T0263821

Cosmetic Dermatology

Guest Editor

VIC A. NARURKAR, MD, FAAD

DERMATOLOGIC CLINICS

www.derm.theclinics.com

Consulting Editor

BRUCE H. THIERS, MD

October 2009 • Volume 27 • Number 4

SAUNDERS an imprint of ELSEVIER, Inc.

W.B. SAUNDERS COMPANY
A Division of Elsevier Inc.

1600 John F. Kennedy Boulevard • Suite 1800 • Philadelphia, PA 19103-2899

http://www.theclinics.com

DERMATOLOGIC CLINICS Volume 27, Number 4
October 2009 ISSN 0733-8635, ISBN-13: 978-1-4377-1209-4, ISBN 10: 1-4377-1209-6

Editor: Carla Holloway
Developmental Editor: Theresa Collier

© **2009 Elsevier ■ All rights reserved.**

This journal and the individual contributions contained in it are protected under copyright by Elsevier, and the following terms and conditions apply to their use:

Photocopying
Single photocopies of single articles may be made for personal use as allowed by national copyright laws. Permission of the Publisher and payment of a fee is required for all other photocopying, including multiple or systematic copying, copying for advertising or promotional purposes, resale, and all forms of document delivery. Special rates are available for educational institutions that wish to make photocopies for non-profit educational classroom use. For information on how to seek permission visit www.elsevier.com/permissions or call: (+44) 1865 843830 (UK)/(+1) 215 239 3804 (USA).

Derivative Works
Subscribers may reproduce tables of contents or prepare lists of articles including abstracts for internal circulation within their institutions. Permission of the Publisher is required for resale or distribution outside the institution. Permission of the Publisher is required for all other derivative works, including compilations and translations (please consult www.elsevier.com/permissions).

Electronic Storage or Usage
Permission of the Publisher is required to store or use electronically any material contained in this journal, including any article or part of an article (please consult www.elsevier.com/permissions). Except as outlined above, no part of this publication may be reproduced, stored in a retrieval system or transmitted in any form or by any means, electronic, mechanical, photocopying, recording or otherwise, without prior written permission of the Publisher.

Notice
No responsibility is assumed by the Publisher for any injury and/or damage to persons or property as a matter of products liability, negligence or otherwise, or from any use or operation of any methods, products, instructions or ideas contained in the material herein. Because of rapid advances in the medical sciences, in particular, independent verification of diagnoses and drug dosages should be made.

Although all advertising material is expected to conform to ethical (medical) standards, inclusion in this publication does not constitute a guarantee or endorsement of the quality or value of such product or of the claims made of it by its manufacturer.

Dermatologic Clinics (ISSN 0733-8635) is published quarterly by Elsevier Inc., 360 Park Avenue South, New York, NY 10010-1710. Months of publication are January, April, July, and October. Business and editorial offices: 1600 John F. Kennedy Blvd., Suite 1800, Philadelphia, PA 19103-2899. Customer service office: 11830 Westline Drive, St. Louis, MO 63146. Periodicals postage paid at New York, NY, and additional mailing offices. Subscription prices are USD 296.00 per year for US individuals, USD 431.00 per year for US institutions, USD 347.00 per year for Canadian individuals, USD 516.00 per year for Canadian institutions, USD 406.00 per year for international individuals, USD 516.00 per year for international institutions, USD 141.00 per year for US students/residents, and USD 204.00 per year for Canadian and international students/residents. International air speed delivery is included in all *Clinics* subscription prices. All prices are subject to change without notice. **POSTMASTER:** Send address changes to *Dermatologic Clinics*, Elsevier Health Sciences Division, Subscription Customer Service, 3251 Riverport Lane, Maryland Heights, MO 63043. **Customer Service: 1-800-654-2452 (U.S. and Canada); 314-447-8871 (outside U.S. and Canada). Fax: 314-447-8029. E-mail: journalscustomerservice-usa@elsevier.com (for print support); journalsonlinesupport-usa@elsevier.com (for online support).**

Reprints. For copies of 100 or more, of articles in this publication, please contact the Commercial Reprints Department, Elsevier Inc., 360 Park Avenue South, New York, New York 10010-1710. Tel.: (212) 633-3813; Fax: (212) 462-1935; Email: repritns@elsevier.com.

The *Dermatologic Clinics* is covered in *MEDLINE/PubMed (Index Medicus)*, *Current Contents/Clinical Medicine*, *Excerpta Medica*, *Chemical Abstracts*, and *ISI/BIOMED*.

Printed and bound by CPI Group (UK) Ltd, Croydon, CR0 4YY
Transferred to Digital Print 2011

Contributors

GUEST EDITOR

VIC A. NARURKAR, MD, FAAD
Chair, Department of Dermatology, California
Pacific Medical Center, San Francisco; Director
and Founder, Bay Area Laser Institute, San
Francisco; and Associate Clinical Professor,
Department of Dermatology, UC Davis School
of Medicine, Sacramento, California

AUTHORS

ROBERT ANOLIK, MD
The Ronald O. Perelman Department
of Dermatology, New York University School
of Medicine, New York, New York

KENNETH BEER, MD, PA
Director, Kenneth Beer MD PA Dermatology, West
Palm Beach and Jupiter; Clinical Instructor in
Dermatology, University of Miami, Miami, Florida;
and Director, The Cosmetic Bootcamp LLC

LEONARD BERNSTEIN, MD
Laser & Skin Surgery Center of New York, New
York, New York

DIANE BERSON, MD
Assistant Clinical Professor, Department
of Dermatology, Weill Cornell Medical College
of Cornell University; and Private Practice,
New York, New York

MELISSA A. BOGLE, MD
Director, The Laser and Cosmetic Surgery Center
of Houston; and Clinical Assistant Professor of
Dermatology, The University of Texas M.D.
Anderson Cancer Center, Houston, Texas

JEREMY A. BRAUER, MD
The Ronald O. Perelman Department
of Dermatology, New York University School
of Medicine, New York, New York

LORI A. BRIGHTMAN, MD
Laser & Skin Surgery Center of New York; and
New York Eye and Ear Infirmary, New York,
New York

JEAN CARRUTHERS, MD
Clinical Professor, Department of Ophthalmology
and Visual Sciences, University of British
Columbia, Vancouver, British Columbia, Canada

ALASTAIR CARRUTHERS, MD
Clinical Professor, Department of Dermatology
and Skin Science, University of British Columbia,
Vancouver, British Columbia, Canada

ANNE CHAPAS, MD
Laser & Skin Surgery Center of New York; and The
Ronald O. Perelman Department of Dermatology,
New York University School of Medicine, New
York, New York

JEFFREY S. DOVER, MD, FRCPC
Director, Skin Care Physicians, Chestnut Hill,
Massachusetts; Associate Clinical Professor
of Dermatology, Section of Dematologic Surgery
and Oncology, Department of Dermatology,
Yale University School of Medicine,
New Haven, Connecticut; Adjunct Professor
of Medicine, Department of Dermatology,
Dartmouth Medical School, Hanover,
New Hampshire

ROY G. GERONEMUS, MD
Director, Laser & Skin Surgery Center of New York; and Clinical Professor of Dermatology, The Ronald O. Perelman Department of Dermatology, New York University School of Medicine, New York, New York

DAVID J. GOLDBERG, MD, JD
Skin Laser & Surgery Specialists of New York and New Jersey; Mount Sinai School of Medicine; and Fordham University School of Law, New York, New York

ELIZABETH HALE, MD
Laser & Skin Surgery Center of New York; and The Ronald O. Perelman Department of Dermatology, New York University School of Medicine, New York, New York

BASIL M. HANTASH, MD, PhD
Instructor, Department of Surgery, Division of Plastic Surgery, Stanford University School of Medicine, Stanford, California

RANELLA HIRSCH, MD, FAAD
Skincare Doctors, Cambridge, Massachusetts

DEREK H. JONES, MD
Skin Care and Laser Physicians of Beverly Hills; and Clinical Assistant Professor of Dermatology, University of California at Los Angeles, Los Angeles, California

JULIE KAREN, MD
Laser & Skin Surgery Center of New York and; The Ronald O. Perelman Department of Dermatology, New York University School of Medicine, New York, New York

MARY P. LUPO, MD
Clinical Professor, Department of Dermatology, Tulane Medical School; and Private Practice Lupo Center for Aesthetic and General Dermatology, New Orleans, Louisiana

VIC A. NARURKAR, MD, FAAD
Chair, Department of Dermatology, California Pacific Medical Center, San Francisco; Director and Founder, Bay Area Laser Institute, San Francisco; and Associate Clinical Professor, Department of Dermatology, UC Davis School of Medicine, Sacramento, California

BOBBY Y. REDDY, MS
Medical Student, Department of Dermatology, New Jersey Medical School, Newark, New Jersey

ANETTA E. RESZKO, MD, PhD
Department of Dermatology, Weill Cornell Medical College of Cornell University, New York, New York

WENDY E. ROBERTS, MD, FAAD
Director, Desert Dermatology Skin Institute, Rancho Mirage, California

AVA T. SHAMBAN, MD, FAAD
Laser Institute of Dermatology and European Skin Care, Santa Monica; and Assistant Clinical Professor, Department of Dermatology, David Geffen School of Medicine at University of California, Los Angeles, California

MEGHAN STIER, BS
Skincare Doctors, Cambridge, Massachusetts

JILL S. WAIBEL, MD
Private Practice, Miami; Volunteer Dermatology Faculty, Department of Dermatology, Miller School of Medicine; and Palm Beach Esthetic Dermatology and Laser Center, West Palm Beach, Florida

ELLIOT WEISS, MD
Laser & Skin Surgery Center of New York, New York, New York

Contents

Cosmeceuticals are topically applied products that are more than merely cosmetic, yet are not true drugs that have undergone rigorous placebo controlled studies for safety and efficacy. There are many review articles that outline the theoretical biologic and clinical actions of these cosmeceuticals and their various ingredients. This article reviews how to incorporate various cosmeceuticals into the treatment regime of patients, depending on the diagnosis and therapies chosen. The practical application of when, why, and on whom to use different products will enable dermatologists to improve the methodology of product selection and, ultimately, improve patient's clinical results.

Since its initial approval by the US Food and Drug Administration (FDA) 20 years ago for the treatment of strabismus, hemifacial spasm, and blepharospasm in adults, botulinum toxin (BTX) has become one of the most frequently requested products in cosmetic rejuvenation around the world. After years of clinical success and consistent safety in the upper face, the use of BTX has expanded and evolved to include increasingly complicated indications. In the hands of adept injectors, the focus has shifted from the treatment of individual dynamic rhytides to shaping, contouring, and sculpting, alone or in combination with other cosmetic procedures, to enhance the aesthetic appearance of the face. Although recent reports have questioned the safety of BTX, 25 years of therapeutic and over 20 years of cosmetic use has demonstrated an impressive record of safety and efficacy when used appropriately by experienced injectors.

Until recently, the use of dermal fillers was limited in the United States by the small number of products approved by the Food and Drug Administration. The products now approved for use in the United States have opened up the range of possibilities for combinations of products that are synergistic in their effects. Combinations of products may be discussed in temporal or anatomic relationships. Temporal combinations refer to the use of different fillers at different times, whereas anatomic combinations refer to the use of different fillers in different parts of the face. Before discussing how the various fillers may be used in combination, it is worthwhile to consider their use in isolation. Soft-tissue augmentation products under consideration in the present article include the hyaluronic acids (HA), poly L lactic acid (PLLA), calcium hydroxylapatite (CAHA), porcine collagen, and silicone.

1980s, the laser-resurfacing industry has produced a multitude of devices employing ablative, nonablative, and fractional ablative technologies. The three approaches largely differ in their method of thermal damage, weighing degrees of efficacy, downtime, and side effect profiles against each other. Nonablative technologies generate some interest, although only for those patient populations seeking mild improvements. Fractional technologies, however, have gained dramatic ground on fully ablative resurfacing. Fractional laser resurfacing, while exhibiting results that fall just short of the ideal outcomes of fully ablative treatments, is an increasingly attractive alternative because of its far more favorable side effect profile, reduced recovery time, and significant clinical outcome.

Results with current skin-tightening technologies are mild to moderate and are not intended to replace surgical procedures. Many patients will choose more subtle tightening to avoid the risks and downtime associated with surgery. Newer treatment protocols have improved treatment predictability and the extent of efficacy, and novel technologies with the potential for even greater results are currently in development. Overall patients' satisfaction can be increased by combining skin tightening with complementary, noninvasive skin treatments, such as botulinum toxin and soft-tissue fillers.

Laser and light-based procedures, fillers, toxins and various peels have revolutionized the field of cosmetic dermatology. With an increasing number of physicians and nonphysicians performing these procedures, and with the availability of a seemingly unlimited array of cosmetic dermatology procedures, the potential for problems and their legal consequences continue to increase. This article will discuss the concept of negligence and the potential for medical malpractice, including the associated problems that may arise when these procedures are performed by physician extenders. The impact of the physician and physician extender relationship, and the legal issues that arise, are also discussed. The article concludes with the legal and ethical issues associated with the promotion of cosmeceutical agents in the field of cosmetic dermatology.

Current aesthetic dermatology rejuvenation options offer minimally invasive, more affordable alternatives to traditional cosmetic surgery. Chemical peels and laser resurfacing can significantly improve the appearance of the skin and stimulate neocollagenesis; botulinum toxin reduces the appearance of dynamic facial lines; and dermal fillers can restore facial fullness. These nonsurgical procedures also carry potential risks. This article reviews potential complications of these procedures and best practices for clinical management to improve outcomes.

Recent advances in technology have drastically improved aesthetic treatment for skin. Of particular interest is the emergence of laser- and lightbased technologies, which have offered great promise among skin-rejuvenation therapies. New laser resurfacing techniques for skin rejuvenation offer significant advantages over conventional ablative lasers, such as the CO_2 and erbiumYAG laser systems. Nonablative and fractional lasers, although not as efficacious as ablative therapies, are associated with significantly diminished complication rates and shortened recovery times. Novel devices combining ablative and fractional technologies have also surfaced, demonstrating noteworthy results. In this review, the authors will discuss the implications of current developments in research and technology for skin rejuvenation. Furthermore, the authors will address emerging therapies for acne vulgaris, lipolysis, and cellulite.

The history of classifying skin types is rather new and there has been considerable progress made with continuing awareness. The Fitzpatrick Skin Phototype Classification remains the gold standard. It is simple and user friendly, however this system fails to accurately predict skin reactions. The Roberts Skin Type Classification System is a tool to predict the skin response to injury and insult from cosmetic procedures and identify the propensity of sequelae from inflammatory skin disorders. It can be a predictor of an impending complication, such as hyperpigmentation and scarring, which can then be avoided. In addition, it includes the skin phototype and photoage. In evaluating patients' skin and developing a cosmetic plan, the four indices outlined in this article, hyper/hypopigmentation risk, scarring risk, skin phototype, and photoage, are crucial to identify for optimal outcomes.

Dermatologic Clinics

THE CLINICS ARE NOW AVAILABLE ONLINE!

Access your subscription at:
www.theclinics.com

Preface

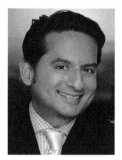

Vic A. Narurkar, MD, FAAD
Guest Editor

Cosmetic dermatology is truly undergoing a renaissance. Just 10 years ago, dermatologists had limited tools in their armamentarium to address the myriad appearance-related issues in the field. The big bang of cosmetic dermatology occurred with the cosmetic use of botulinum toxins. This addressed one of the four *R*s in global rejuvenation—*r*elaxation of muscles of facial expression. The use of botulinum toxins has grown from merely addressing glabellar rhytids to the sophisticated use in facial shaping. The rapid development of dermal fillers soon exploded, addressing the second *R*—*r*efilling of loss of facial and nonfacial volume. For the majority of the twentieth century, dermal fillers were limited to collagens and the concept of filling in lines. The explosion of varieties of classes of fillers now enables dermatologists to achieve facial sculpting. The expansion of selective photothermolysis led to the development of a multitude of devices addressing the third *R*—*r*esurfacing the facial and nonfacial canvas. The initial energy-based devices were often bulky and slow, with limited applications. Technologic advances in energy-based devices have made them more portable, ergonomic, and, most recently, even available for home use. The development of cosmeceuticals and skin care products completes the fourth *R*—*r*etention of skin elements. In addition to more sophisticated materials, enhanced delivery systems of these cosmeceuticals are making them more effective. These advances have paralleled increased global awareness, with the development of new skin-typing classification systems to address the complexities of ethnicity, response of skin to injury, and photodamage. We are now able to treat global skin with greater safety and efficacy. Finally, combination therapies are being used for global nonsurgical restoration—off and on face—using toxins, fillers, devices, and skin care in synergy. As we enter the new millennium, the field continues to grow at lightning speed. This issue of *Dermatologic Clinics* reviews current and emerging technologies in the field of cosmetic dermatology.

Vic A. Narurkar, MD, FAAD
Department of Dermatology
University of California Davis School of Medicine
Sacramento, CA 95817, USA

E-mail address:
info@bayarealaserdr.com (V.A. Narurkar)

Dermatol Clin 27 (2009) xi
doi:10.1016/j.det.2009.09.001
0733-8635/09/$ – see front matter © 2009 Elsevier Inc. All rights reserved.

Cosmeceuticals: Practical Applications

Anetta E. Reszko, MD, PhD[a],*, Diane Berson, MD[a,b],
Mary P. Lupo, MD[c]

KEYWORDS

- Antioxidants • Cosmeceuticals
- Procedure protocols • Vitamins • Pigment-lightening
- Anti-inflammatory • Peptides

Cosmeceutical is a term coined approximately 2 decades ago by Albert Kligman to refer to topically applied products that are not merely cosmetics that adorn or camouflage, yet are not true drugs that have undergone rigorous placebo-controlled studies for safety and efficacy.[1] This continues to be an area of new product development, with an ever-growing marketplace as baby boomers continue to age. There are many review articles that outline the theoretical biologic and clinical actions of these cosmeceuticals and their various ingredients.[2–7] This article reviews how to incorporate various cosmeceuticals into the treatment regime of patients, depending on the diagnosis and treatment chosen. The practical application of when, why, and on whom to use different products will enable dermatologists to improve the methodology of product selection and, ultimately, improve patient's clinical results.

Cosmeceuticals can be divided into 7 main product categories (**Box 1**).

In choosing an effective cosmeceuticals regimen it is critical to match patients and their problems with the appropriate products. Most patients have multiple needs, and they should be matched with products that offer ingredients with multifactorial benefits.

Certain treatment principles apply to all therapeutic protocols. Morning treatment protocols should provide environmental (antioxidant, sunscreen, sun block) and antimicrobial protection whereas evening/night protocols should be centered on tissue repair (retinoid).

This article highlights several common diagnoses and discusses how and which cosmeceuticals should help, or at least compliment, procedures or prescriptions. Furthermore, the use of cosmeceuticals in conjunction with commonly performed office-based procedures, such as chemical peels, microdermabrasion, photorejuvenation, and laser resurfacing, is discussed.

MELASMA
Introduction

Even skin pigmentation is considered to be a universal sign of youth and beauty. Pigmentary alterations seen in melasma are sharply demarcated, brown patches, typically located on the malar prominences and forehead. Three clinically apparent patterns are centrofacial, malar, and mandibular (rare). Melasma is more frequent in higher skin types (III, IV, and V) and is especially prominent among Asian and Hispanic people. The pigment deposition in melasma is epidermally or dermally based, with most cases showing both.

Treatment of melasma is often difficult and might require multiple treatment modalities. Sunlight protection with a broad-spectrum sunscreen with ultraviolet A (UVA) and ultraviolet B (UVB) coverage is the cornerstone of the therapy, because UVB, UVA, and visible light are

[a] Department of Dermatology, Weill Cornell Medical College of Cornell University, 1305 York Avenue, 9th Floor, New York, New York 10021, USA
[b] Private Practice, 211 East 53 Street, New York, New York 10022, USA
[c] Department of Dermatology, Tulane Medical School, Private Practice Lupo Center for Aesthetic and General Dermatology, 145 Robert E Lee Boulevard, Suite 302, New Orleans, LA 70124, USA
* Corresponding author.
E-mail address: anetta.reszko@gmail.com (A.E. Reszko).

Dermatol Clin 27 (2009) 401–416
doi:10.1016/j.det.2009.08.005
0733-8635/09/$ – see front matter © 2009 Elsevier Inc. All rights reserved.

Box 1
Cosmeceuticals product categories

- Sunscreen
- Antioxidant
- Anti-inflammatory
- Pigment lightening
- Collagen repair
- Exfoliation
- Hydration/barrier repair

all capable of stimulating melanogenesis. Sunscreens and sun blockers containing physical blockers, such as titanium dioxide and zinc oxide, are preferable to chemical blockers because of their broader protection.

The mainstay of treatment of melasma is topical depigmenting agents (**Box 2**).

In addition, retinoids, exfoliation with superficial chemical peels, mechanical dermabrasion, or non-ablative (intense pulsed light [IPL]) or fractional microablative technologies may provide added benefit. Combination therapy centers on the fact that if melanogenesis is inhibited (depigmenting agents) and keratinocyte turnover is increased (chemical peels, retinoids, lasers/IPL), the time to clinical improvement can be reduced.

Pigment Modifying Agents

Currently available pigment lightening products target individual stages of melanogenesis or block melanin transfer from melanocytes to keratinocytes. The following are commercially available, highly effective pigment lightening preparations.

Hydroquinone

Hydroquinone (HQ), benzene-1,4-diol, is an inhibitor of melanogenesis by (1) inhibiting tyrosinase, and (2) a direct melanocyte cytotoxic effect. HQ is a poor substrate of tyrosinase, competing for

Box 2
Pigment modifying agents

Hydroquinone

Kojic acid

Vitamins C and E

Azelaic acid

Ellagic acid (polyphenol)

Pycnogenol

Fatty acids (linoloic acid)

Niacinamide (B3)

Soy (STI)

tyrosine oxidation in active melanocytes. The cytotoxic effect of HQ is mediated by reversible inhibition of DNA and RNA synthesis.

Clinical improvement with over-the-counter 2% HQ as monotherapy is usually seen in 4 to 6 weeks, with improvement approaching a plateau at 4 months. Because of its irritant properties and increased risk of postinflammatory hyperpigmentation (PIH), HQ is often combined with topical medium potency steroids. Compounded HQ is available in the United States as Tri-Luma (Galderma, Fort Worth, Texas; 0.01% fluocinolone, 4% HQ and 0.05% tretinoin) in a cream formulation.[5]

In recent years, the use of HQ has become a subject of marked controversy, that led to its removal from markets in Europe and in parts of Asia.[5] In recent months, the Food and Drug Administration (FDA) voiced concerns about the safety of HQ for topical application. The basis for the FDA's concern was the increasing number of reports of ochronosis, (bluish-black discoloration) of HQ topically treated sites,[8] and reports of potential carcinogenicity of systemic HQ. The mechanism of HQ-induced ochronosis remains unknown. It is usually observed in patients of African descent who have been treated with high concentrations of HQ for several years. Histologically, the initial stages of ochronosis are characterized by the degeneration of collagen and elastic fibers. In later stages, ochronotic deposits are seen, consisting of crescent-shaped, ochre-colored fibers in the dermis. It is unclear whether HQ itself, high concentrations of HQ, or other substances that exist in the topical preparations contribute to the onset of ochronosis.

The carcinogenic properties of HQ were demonstrated in rodent models following systemic administration of high quantities of HQ. The human potential for carcinogenicity has not been demonstrated. Nonetheless, because of the rapid uptake and distribution of HQ applied to the skin, it has been speculated that the risks of topical application are similar to, or greater than, those of pulmonary or gastrointestinal exposure.[9] With topical application, the first-pass liver metabolism of HQ is circumvented and HQ, a benzene derivate, can reach systemic circulation without prior detoxification.

Azelaic acid

Azelaic acid is a naturally occurring, saturated 9-carbon dicarboxylic acid derived from *Pityrosporum ovale*. It is a weak competitive inhibitor of tyrosinase. Azelaic acid also exhibits antiproliferative and cytotoxic effects on melanocytes via inhibition of thioredoxin reductase, an enzyme involved in mitochondrial oxidoreductase activation and DNA synthesis. Unlike HQ, azelaic acid seems to target only abnormally hyperactive melanocytes, and thus will not lighten skin with normally functioning melanocytes. Thus, the benefits of azelaic acid might extend beyond the realm of cosmetic medicine, as it may play a role in preventing development of, or in therapy for, lentigo maligna and lentigo maligna melanoma.[5,6]

The clinical efficacy and pigment lightening properties of azelaic acid have been studied in large groups of diverse skin types, including skin types III to VI, and its efficacy has been compared with that of 4% HQ cream, although with a slightly higher rate of local irritation.[10,11] Azelaic acid is commercially available as a topical 20% cream. The primary adverse effect of topical application is skin irritation. For added benefit, azelaic acid may be combined with 15–20% glycolic acid (GA).

Niacinamide

Niacinamide, also known as nicotinamide, is a water-soluble component of the vitamin B complex group. In vivo, nicotinamide is incorporated into nicotinamide adenine dinucleotide (NAD) and nicotinamide adenine dinucleotide phosphate (NADP), coenzymes essential for enzymatic oxidation reduction reactions, including tissue mitochondrial respiration and lipid metabolism.

Niacinamide inhibits melanine transfer to keratinocyte. Bissett and colleagues[12–15] showed that niacinamide reduced the appearance of hyperpigmented macules, fine lines and wrinkles, red blotchiness, skin sallowness, and increased skin elasticity. In addition, niacinamide helped alleviate some of the symptoms of rosacea by increasing hydration, reducing transepidermal water loss, and improving the barrier function of the stratum corneum.

Kojic acid

Kojic acid, 5-hydroxymethyl-4H-pyrane-4-one, is a hydrophilic fungal derivative derived from *Aspergillus* and *Penicillium* species, exerting its biologic activity by inhibiting copper binding to tyrosinase. It is one of the most commonly used over-the-counter skin lightening agents sold worldwide. Albeit Kojic acid was recently removed from the market in Japan due its sensitizing properties.

Licorice extract

Licorice (*Glycyrrhiza glabra, Glycyrrhiza inflate*) extract has been used as a natural remedy for centuries for its anti-inflammatory and anti-irritant properties. Licorice extract derived from the root of *Glycyrrhiza glabra*, glabridin, has dual pigment modulating and anti-inflammatory properties. Active ingredients in licorice extract are the flavenoids, liquirtin and isoliquertin. Licorice extract leads to skin lightening primarily by dispersing melanin.[16] In cultured B16 melanoma cells, glabridin inhibits tyrosinase activity without affecting DNA synthesis rates.[17] Topical application of glabridin has been shown to reduce UVB-induced pigmentation and erythema in the skin of guinea pigs. In vitro anti-inflammatory effects of glabridin relate to inhibition of superoxide production and activity of cyclooxygenase.[17]

For clinical efficacy, glabridin must be applied at a dosage of 1 g/d for at least 4 weeks. Licorice extract is considered a weak lightening agent and must be combined with other agents for optimal clinical results.

Arbutin and deoxyarbutin

Derived from the leaves of the *Vaccinium vitisidaea*, arbutin is a gluconopyranoside that inhibits tyrosinase. It also inhibits melanosome maturation without associated melanocyte toxicity.[18] Arbutin at a concentration of 3% is available in Japan in several over-the-counter preparations. Higher concentrations may provide additional therapeutic benefit, but paradoxic darkening may occur. Deoxyarbutin is a synthetically modified derivative of arbutin with enhanced pigment lightening properties.[19]

Aloesin

Aloesis is a low-molecular-weight glycoprotein derived from the aloe vera plant. It functions through the competitive inhibition of tyrosinase at the dihydroxyphenylalanine (DOPA) oxidation site.[20–22] Therapeutic application of aloesin is limited by its hydrophilic nature and inability to penetrate the skin.

Edelweiss complex

Edelweiss complex is a new approach targeting skin discoloration. It relies on antisense oligonucleotides that block targeted gene transcription and modulate melanogenesis. This technology offers unique specificity, biologic stability, and safety in whitening of all skin types. In a clinical study of 30 Asian patients with dyschromia of the hands, the test product applied twice daily for 8 weeks significantly whitened hyperpigmented and normal skin.[23]

Vitamin C

Numerous studies have confirmed the beneficial effects of systemic (oral and intravenous [IV] administration[24]) and topically applied ascorbic acid (vitamin C) in the treatment of melasma.[5,25,26] In a randomized, split-face clinical trial 16 women were treated with a nightly application of 5%

ascorbic acid cream on one side of the face and 4% HQ cream on the opposite side, for 16 weeks.

The HQ and ascorbic acid treated sides had good and excellent results in 93% and 62.5% of patients, respectively. Colorimetric measures showed no statistical differences. Topically applied ascorbic acid was well tolerated with low rates of side effects reported (6.2% vs 68.7% in HQ group).[26]

Vitamin C can also be combined with other treatment modalities such as trichloroacetic acid (TCA) peel for synergistic effect.[25] One limitation of topically applied ascorbic acid is its inherent instability (for a detailed discussion see section on Rosacea).

Retinoids

Retinoids are synthetic and natural compounds with structure and activity similar to that of vitamin A. Vitamin A exists as retinol (a vitamin A alcohol), retinal (a vitamin A aldehyde, and retinoic acid (a vitamin A acid). All these forms are interconvertible. Biologic activity of retinoids relates to their ability to activate RAR $\alpha\beta\gamma$ and RXR $\alpha\beta\gamma$ receptors, and increases from retinol to retinaldehyde to retinoic acid.

A plethora of prescription and over-the-counter retinoids exist. Topical retinoid's ability to depigment is based on its ability to disperse melanosomes, interfere with melanocyte-keratinocyte pigment transfer, and accelerate epidermal turnover and, subsequently, pigment loss.[27,28] In addition, retinoids may inhibit melanogenesis by inhibiting tyrosinase and DOPAchrome conversion factor.[29]

Topical tretinoin (*trans*-retinoic acid) can be effective in the treatment of melasma as monotherapy. In a large-scale, double-blind, placebo-controlled study of 50 white women, topical 0.1% tretinoin caused a marked clinical improvement, 68% and 5% for tretinoin and placebo groups, respectively, at 40 weeks. Clinical improvement was consistent with calorimetric and histologic assessment.[30] Epidermal pigment was reduced by 36% in the tretinoin-treated group.

Overall, the response to tretinoin treatment is less than with HQ and can be slow, with improvement seen after 6 months or longer. Tretinoin as a monotherapy is not an approved treatment of melasma. Nonetheless, a forementioned combination regimen of tretinoin, HQ, and a topical corticosteroid (fluocinolone acetonide) is FDA approved and commercially available as Tri-Luma.[29]

The major adverse effect of retinoids is skin irritation, especially when the more effective, higher concentrations are used. Temporary photosensitivity and paradoxic hyperpigmentation can also occur.

Chemical Peels, Microdermabrasion, Nonablative and Fractional Ablative Light, and Laser Technologies

Chemical peels (superficial peels, including 20%–30% salicylic acid, 30%–40% GA, β-lipohydroxy acid [LHA]), microdermabrasion, and nonablative and fractional ablative technologies[31,32] have been used extensively for the treatment of melasma. Periprocedural use of appropriate cosmeceuticals may enhance postprocedural healing and their continued use may extend the duration of treatment benefits.

A few general principles apply. First, a thorough medical history, including any hypertrophic scarring, viral (herpetic), bacterial (*Staphylococcus*), and yeast infections, must be obtained. Appropriate antiviral, antibacterial, and antiyeast treatments should be initiated immediately before, and continued for 7 to 10 days following the treatment to prevent infection, as cutaneous infection in the immediate postsurgical period might lead to significant PIH and possible scarring. All medications should be known and oral contraceptives and known photosensitizers should be discontinued if medically possible. Second, medium to high potency topical fluorinated steroids administered 2 to 3 days before treatment and continued for up to 1 to 2 weeks after the treatment might lead to decreased swelling and bleeding. Third, all medications that increase the risk of bleeding (eg, aspirin, nonsteroidal anti-inflammatories, vitamin E, ginkgo) should be stopped unless medically necessary. Fourth, to minimize the risk of scarring and PIH, retinoids or chemical peels should be stopped 3 days (superficial chemical peels) to 2 weeks (nonablative, fractional ablative resurfacing) before the procedure. Systemic isotretinoin should be stopped within 6 (nonablative) to 12 (fractional ablative and ablative) months of the procedure. Fifth, dark-skinned or tanned individuals are at higher risk of postinflammatory dyschromia. The risk of postinflammatory dyschromia after fractional resurfacing may be minimized by pretreatment with HQ.[31]

Postprocedure patients may resume preoperative treatment regimens including depigmenting agents. Following nonablative procedures and fractional ablative procedures, depigmenting agents may be initiated after 1 to 2 weeks or at the first sign of hyperpigmentation. Use of emollients, gentle skin care with toners, and mild cleansers and sun blocks is crucial for optimal healing in the immediate postoperative period.

Laser treatments with Q-switched lasers (neodymium:yttrium-aluminum-garnet [Nd:YAG], frequency-doubled [532 nm] and nonfrequency-doubled [1064 nm]), ruby laser (694 nm), and ablative carbon dioxide and erbium:YAG (2940 nm), seem to show limited usefulness in the treatment of melasma, with high rates of melasma recurrence and a high incidence of PIH.[29]

Recently, fractional resurfacing with a 1550-nm erbium:glass laser (Fraxel SR 750, Reliant Technologies, Inc, Mountain View, CA) has proved to be a promising treatment modality with marked postprocedural clinical, histologic, and ultrastructural improvement.[32–34]

Microdermabrasion

In a large study of 533 patients with melasma, Kunachak and colleagues[35] reported a melasma clearance rate of 97% after microdermabrasion at long-term follow-up. PIH and postprocedural hyperemia were responsive to 3% to 5% topical HQ or 0.1% triamcinolone.

Chemical Peels

Salicylic acid
Grimes[36] reported moderate to significant improvement of melasma in 4 of 6 patients with skin types V and VI, treated with a series of 20% to 30% salicylic acid (SA) peels (every 2 weeks) plus HQ (administered for 2 weeks before initiation of SA series). The treatment protocol was well tolerated with no reported postinflammatory dyschromia. SA peels without pretreatment with HQ were associated with higher risk of hyperpigmentation (Diane Berson, MD, unpublished observation, personal communication, 2008).

GA
The usefulness of serial GA (an α hydroxyl acid) peels (increasing concentrations 35%, 50%, and 70%) with topical therapy with azaleic acid and adapalene was studied in 28 women with recalcitrant melasma.[37] The combination therapy (GA peels, retinoid, and azaleic acid) group had superior clinical improvement compared with the retinoid plus azaleic acid group. Combined treatment with serial GA peels, azelaic acid cream, and adapalene gel may be an effective and safe therapy for recalcitrant melasma.

Lim and Tham[38] conducted a 26-week, single-blind, split-face study of 10 Asian women treated with GA peels ranging in concentration from 20% to 70%, administered every 3 weeks alone or in combination with topical HQ plus 10% GA. The best clinical improvement was noted in women treated with the combination therapy, although results did not reach statistical significance.

ROSACEA
Introduction

Rosacea is a common, chronic skin disorder that primarily affects the central and convex areas of the face. The nose, cheeks, chin, forehead, and glabella are the most frequently affected sites. The disease has a variety of clinical manifestations ranging from flushing, persistent erythema, telangiectasias, papules, pustules, tissue hyperplasia, and sebaceous gland hyperplasia. Diagnosis of rosacea is based primarily on clinically recognizable morphologic characteristics. An expert committee assembled by the National Rosacea Society on the Classification and Staging of Rosacea defined and classified rosacea in April 2002 into 4 clinical subtypes based primarily on morphologic characteristics. The subtypes include erythematotelangiectatic rosacea, papulopustular rosacea, phymatous rosacea, and ocular rosacea. The pathogenesis of rosacea is complex, with genetic and vascular elements, climatic exposures, matrix degeneration, chemicals and ingested agents, pilosebaceous unit abnormalities, and microbial organisms likely playing a role.[39]

FDA approved rosacea treatment options include systemic and topical antibiotics with antimicrobial and anti-inflammatory properties, azelaic acid, and topical immunomodulators. These medical therapy options are often insufficient, especially for erythematotelangiectatic rosacea motivating patients to search for alternative herbal anti-inflammatories and botanicals. "Anti-red" cosmeceuticals can be combined with prescription medications and in-office procedures.

Anti-inflammatory Botanicals

Licochalcone A (licorice extract)
Licorice extract has marked anti-inflammatory properties. In in vitro studies, licochalcone A isolated from the roots of *Glycyrrhiza inflate* suppresses inflammation via indirect inhibition of the cyclooxygenase (COX) and lipoxygenase pathways. Licochalcone A in vivo decreases UVB-induced erythema, reduces proinflammatory cytokines, and UVB-induced prostaglandin E2 (PGE_2) release by keratinocytes.[17,40] In an 8-week clinical trial of 32 women with mild to moderate rosacea and 30 women with facial erythema, application of 4 test products containing licochalcone A (cleanser, moisturizer with sun protection factor [SPF] 15, spot concealer, and

night moisturizing cream) resulted in a significant reduction of erythema at 4 and 8 weeks after initiation of treatment (7% vs 23%, respectively). Licochalcone A-containing cosmeceuticals were well tolerated for everyday use.[40] In another study, topical application of a licochalcone A-containing extract twice daily for 3 days resulted in a significant reduction in UV-induced and shaving-induced erythema.[41]

Azelaic acid
Topical azelaic acid is an FDA approved treatment of rosacea and acne vulgaris and is useful for acne-induced PIH.[42]

Aloe vera
Aloe vera has been widely used in traditional medicine to accelerate healing of wounds and burns. The active ingredients of aloe vera include SA (antimicrobial and anti-inflammatory properties via inhibition of thromboxane and prostaglandin synthesis), magnesium lactate (antipruritic properties via inhibition of histidine decarboxylase), and gel polysaccharides (anti-inflammatory activity by immunomodulation).[43]

The anti-inflammatory properties and clinical efficacy of aloe vera were tested in a double-blind, placebo-controlled trial of 60 patients with mild to moderate psoriasis.[44] Treatment 3 times daily for 5 consecutive days per week for a maximum of 4 weeks with 0.5% aloe vera cream resulted in clearing of psoriatic plaques in 83% of patients compared with only 8% of the placebo group.

Chamomile
Chamomile (*Matricaria recutita*) has long been used in traditional folk medicine for the treatment of skin irritation and atopic dermatitis. The active components of chamomile include α-bis-abolol, α-bis-abolol oxide A and B, and matricin,[45] all of which are potent inhibitors of COX and lipoxygenase pathways. Chamomile also contains the flavonoids apigenin, luteolin, and quercetin, all potent inhibitors of histamine release.[45] In the skin of healthy volunteers, the anti-inflammatory properties of topical chamomile were comparable with approximately 60% of that produced by hydrocortisone 0.025% cream application.[46]

Feverfew
Feverfew (*Tanacetum parthenium*) is a nonsteroidal anti-inflammatory agent with marked anti-irritant and antioxidant properties. Anti-inflammatory properties of feverfew include inhibition of pro-inflammatory cytokine (tumor necrosis factor α [TNFα], interferon-γ [INF-γ], interleukin-2 [IL-2], IL-4) release, decrease in nuclear factor κB (NF-κB) mediated gene transcription, inhibition of neutrophil chemotaxis, and inhibition of adhesion molecule expression.[47] One drawback of topical application of feverfew is a high potential for topical sensitization and irritation. Newly developed purified feverfew extract (Feverfew, PFE) retains the anti-inflammatory properties of feverfew with minimal skin sensitization.

The anti-inflammatory properties of feverfew, as assessed by inhibition of TNFα release, seem to be far superior to other botanicals including teas (green, black, white), echinacea, licorice extract, chamomile, and aloe vera.[47] In a 4-week, controlled, full-face clinical trial, 35 women with mild to moderate facial rosacea were treated with a moisturizing agent containing PFE with an SPF of 15, and a nightly moisturizing cream with PFE, once daily. At 4 weeks, marked improvement in erythema, tactile surface roughness, visual dryness, and overall facial irritation was noted. Application of the feverfew was well tolerated.[4,47] PFE was also shown to reduce UVB-induced erythema in a normal skin. Skin treated for 2 days with 1% PFE and exposed to increasing minimal erythema doses (MEDs; 0.5, 1, 1.5 MED) of UVB showed a marked reduction of erythema at 24 and 48 hours compared with untreated control at all MEDs tested.[48]

Oatmeal
Oatmeal is one of a limited number of natural compounds recognized and regulated by the FDA. Colloidal oatmeal, dehulled oats ground to a fine powder, is recognized by the FDA as a skin protectant that, in addition to providing temporary skin protection, relieves minor pruritus and irritation caused by eczema, rashes, poison ivy, and other contact allergens and insect bites.[49] Colloidal oatmeal has a combination of components and properties well suited for the treatment of inflammatory skin conditions. It cleanses, moisturizes, provides barrier protection, and exhibits anti-inflammatory activity.

The antioxidant constituents of oats are avenanthramides, which are polyphenolic compounds. Isolated avenanthramides reduce proinflammatory cytokines (IL-8) and transcription factors (NF-κB) in cultured human keratinocytes,[50] reduce histamine-induced pruritus in humans, and decrease UVB-induced erythema. In recent months, a topical formulation of proprietary standardized avenanthramide became commercially available as *Avena sativa* kernel.

Pycnogenol
Pycnogenol is a standardized extract from French maritime pine bark (*Pinus pinaster*). The extract's active ingredients include proanthocyanidins,

shown to have photoprotective, antimicrobial, antioxidant, anti-inflammatory, and anticarcinogenic effects.[51,52] Its anti-inflammatory properties may include the inhibition of INF-γ and down-regulation of expression of interstitial cell adhesion molecule 1 (ICAM-1) on the surface of keratinocytes. Pycnogenol also converts the vitamin C radical to its active form and raises levels of glutathione and other free-radical scavengers.[3,53] In an animal model, topical application of 0.05% to 0.2% Pycnogenol reduced ultraviolet radiation (UVR)-induced erythema, inflammation, and tumor carcinogenesis in a dose-dependent manner.[52] In a clinical trial of healthy volunteers, 8-week-long oral Pycnogenol supplementation reduced UV-induced erythema.[54]

Lycopene

Lycopene, a carotinoid, exhibits considerable reductive potential and antioxidant activity.[55] When applied topically before UVA exposure, it prevents apoptosis, reduces inflammation, and diminishes expression of enzymes implicated in carcinogenesis.[56] In addition, lycopene has the ability to regenerate vitamin E (α-tocopherol).[55] The clinical usefulness of lycopene still remains to be proved. In a clinical trial of 10 volunteers, 6% topical lycopene cream reduced UV-induced erythema to a greater extent than a topical mixture of vitamin C and vitamin E.[55] In an in vitro study on human fibroblasts exposed to UVA radiation, lycopene offered photoprotection and reduced UVA-induced levels of matrix metalloprotease 1 (MMP-1) only when combined with vitamin E.[56]

Silymarin

Silymarin, a polyphenolic flavonoid from the milk thistle plant, *Silybum marianum*, inhibits lipoprotein oxidation and acts as a free-radical scavenger.[57] In animal models, silymarin showed chemoprotective and anticarcinogenic acitivity.[57,58] It reduced UVB radiation-induced erythema, edema, and keratinocyte apoptosis through the inhibition of inflammatory cytokines and pyrimidine dimers.[59,60] Clinically, silymarin alleviates the symptoms of rosacea. In a double-blinded, placebo-controlled study of 46 patients with rosacea, topical application of silymarin and methylsulfonilmethane for 1 month resulted in statistically significant improvements in erythema, papules, pruritus, and skin hydration.[61]

Quercetin

Found in many fruits and vegetables, the flavonoid quercetin has antioxidant and anti-inflammatory properties. Its anti-inflammatory activity results from inhibition of the enzymatic actions of lipooxygenase and COX-2, and from blocking histamine release. Quercetin also enhances tumor cell apoptosis.[3] In a mouse model, quercetin reduced UVA-induced oxidative stress.[62] In vitro quercetin inhibited growth of melanoma cells.[63]

Allantoin

Allantoin derived from the comfrey root has anti-inflammatory and antioxidant effects. It has been shown to repair cutaneous photodamage and reduce inflammation following UVR exposure.[64]

Chemical Peels

Chemical peels, β-hydroxy acids and α-hydroxy acids (GA) are widely used for the treatment of acne rosacea. Clinical experience has long shown effectiveness of SA in the treatment of acne rosacea. SA targets comedonal and inflammatory lesions and has better sustained efficacy and fewer side effects than GA peels.[65,66]

Lee and colleagues[67] reported improvement in acne in 35 Korean patients treated with 30% SA peels. Grimes[36] reported moderate clearing of inflammatory acne lesions in 8 of 9 dark-skinned patients (diverse ethnicity including subjects of Asian, African, and Hispanic descent) treated with a series of 20% to 30% SA peels with 4% HQ pretreatment. This treatment regimen facilitated resolution of PIH, and a decrease in overall pigmentation of the face.

An SA derivative, lipohydroxyacid (LHA) (commercially available in concentrations up to 10%) has recently been introduced in the United States. With an additional fatty chain, LHA has increased lipophilicity that allows for efficient exfoliation, and increased antibacterial, anti-inflammatory, antifungal, and anticomedogenic properties even at low concentrations.[68] Studies have shown strong keratinolytic properties with good penetration through the epidermis and into the pilosebaceous unit.

In a randomized, controlled clinical trial, Uhoda and colleagues[69] studied LHA peels in acne-prone women and women with comedonal acne. UV light video recordings and computerized image analysis showed significantly decreased numbers and sizes of microcomedones and a reduction in the density of follicular keratotic plugs in the LHA treated group.

Laser Therapy and IPL

Laser therapy with pulsed dye lasers (PDL 585-595 nm), potassium-titanyl-phosphate (KTP), and IPL for acne rosacea has been used extensively for the reduction of telangiectasias, erythema, flushing, and improving skin texture.[70,71] The primary mode of action of laser/ILP therapy is selective photothermolysis of telangiectatic superficial blood vessels.

In a recent small pilot study of 10 rosacea patients treated with either IPL or PDL, 5 patients (3 after IPL and 2 after PDL) had lower levels of cathelicidin, an antimicrobial peptide. Cathelicidins were recently shown to play a central role in the pathogenesis of rosecea.[72] In addition to directly mediating antimicrobial activity, cathelicidins have the potential to trigger the immune host tissue response by promoting leukocyte chemotaxis, angiogenesis, and the expression of components of the extracellular matrix.[73] Patients with rosacea express higher levels of cathelicidins peptides in affected facial areas compared with similar anatomic regions of unaffected controls.

Although the results of the aforementioned trial did not reach statistical significance, the study raised an interesting mechanism for clinical improvement of rosacea symptoms after IPL or laser treatment.[74] Natural anti-inflammatory agents could potentially limit the cathelicidin-medicated inflammatory cascade.

PHOTOAGING (RHYTIDS AND DYSCHROMIA)
Introduction

In the treatment of aging skin, a new generation of cosmeceuticals offers clinical benefits. Ultrapotent antioxidants, stem cell modulators, and antisense DNA technologies are advancing our clinical understanding of the intrinsic and extrinsic aging processes, offering targeted strategies for slowing down or reversing the signs of aging. The aging process has intrinsic and extrinsic bases. These 2 clinically and biologically independent and distinct processes affect skin structure and function.

Intrinsic or innate aging is a naturally occurring process that occurs from slow, but progressive and irreversible, tissue degeneration. Telomere shortening and metabolic oxidative damage with free reactive oxygen species (ROS) generation all play a role in the innate aging process.[75] Based on a unique genetic imprint, intrinsic aging affects everyone at different rates. On a histologic level, intrinsic aging is characterized by decreased collagen synthesis, degeneration of elastic fiber networks, and loss of hydration. Clinically, fine wrinkling of the skin, loss of skin tone, skin laxity, and loss of subcutaneous fat occur.

Of the extrinsic factors, UV and infrared (IR) radiation, environmental pollutants, and physical factors (cold, wind) play a crucial role. UVA radiation is the prime driver of premature aging. Clinically, extrinsic photoaging is characterized by coarse wrinkling and furrowing with an apparent thickening of the skin, elastosis, and a variety of benign, premalignant, and malignant neoplasms.[76] Histologically, photodamaged skin shows a 20% decrease in total collagen and decreased cellular content compared with sun-protected skin.[77] Moreover, pigmentary alterations and telangiectasias contribute to an aged appearance by creating shadows and areas of contrast on the face.

Antioxidants

Antioxidants have long been used in the cosmetic industry for their multifaceted benefits, offering antiaging and anti-inflammatory properties. In addition, antioxidants confer a degree of photoprotection and anticarcinogenesis by quenching free-radical species generated by cellular metabolism and direct exposure to UV radiation. They also block UV-induced inflammatory pathways.

Tea
Tea (black, green, white, oolong) is derived from the leaves and buds of the tea plant (*Camellia sinensis*). Different varieties of tea result from differential processing, oxidation, and fermentation of the tea leaves and buds.[78] Active ingredients in tea include polyphenolic catechins such as epicatechin, epicatechin-3-gallate (ECG), epigallocatechin (EGC), and epigallocatechin-3-gallate (EGCG).[4]

Green tea offers antioxidant, anti-inflammatory, and anticarcinogenic properties with systemic and topical administration.[79] Early studies on hairless mice fed green tea showed a dose-dependent reduction of UV-induced carcinogenesis.[80,81] Similar anticarcinogenic and chemoprotective effects were shown after topical application of green tea polyphenolic catechins (GTP) in mice. GTP is the active ingredient in green tea and limits UV-induced redness, the number of sunburn cells, collagen, and cellular DNA damage.[81]

In healthy volunteers, topical GTP (EGCG and ECG) inhibited UV-induced erythema and reduced formation of cyclobutane pyrimidine dimers, a marker of DNA damage.[82,83] Green tea has also has been studied for use in cosmetic applications. In a clinical study of 40 women with moderate photoaging, Chin and colleagues found increased elastic tissue content in the skin of women treated with 300 mg of green tea supplements twice daily and topical 10% green tea cream daily. Histologic improvement nonetheless did not correlate with clinical improvement after 8 weeks of treatment, suggesting that (1) histologic improvement (especially mild to moderate) may not translate into short-term clinical improvement, and (2) clinical correlation of all histologic findings is essential.[84]

Vitamin C, vitamin E, and ferulic acid

Cosmeceutical preparations of vitamins C (L-ascorbic acid) and E (D-alpha-tocopherol) play a major role in the treatment of photoaged skin. In vivo, vitamin C blocks UVR-induced erythema. In vitro, vitamin C stimulates fibroblasts, increases rates of neocollagenesis, decreases melanin formation, and exhibits anti-inflammatory activity. The effects of cutaneous vitamin C application were evaluated in a double-blind, half-face trial. A 12-week treatment with vitamin C complex consisting of 10% ascorbic acid (water soluble) and 7% tetrahexyldecyl ascorbate (lipid soluble provitamin C) resulted in significant improvement in photoaging scores and skin wrinkling. Histologic analysis revealed increased collagen content in sites treated with vitamin C complex.[85]

Diet is the sole source of vitamin C in humans. Gastrointestinal absorption is the rate-limiting factor in cutaneous delivery of vitamin C. Therefore, even supraphysiologic doses of vitamin C through oral administration do not increase the cutaneous concentration to optimal levels. Exposure to sunlight and environmental pollutants deplete cutaneous vitamin C. Even minimal UV exposure of 1.6 times the MED decreases the level of vitamin C to 70% of the normal level. Exposure to 10 ppm of ozone in city pollution decreases the level of epidermal vitamin C by 55%.[79]

Vitamin E is the most important lipid soluble, membrane-bound antioxidant in plasma, cellular membranes, and tissues. Similar to vitamin C, vitamin E is supplied solely through diet. In animal studies, vitamin E, decreases the rate of UVR-induced tumor formation. In clinical studies, topically applied vitamin E decreased the appearance of wrinkles, solar lentigines, and overall photoaging.

In tissues, vitamins C and E act synergistically to provide antioxidant protection. When used in combination, topical L-ascorbic acid (15%) and D-α-tocopherol (1%) resulted in a fourfold greater protection against UV-induced erythema, compared with a twofold increase with either agent alone.

The inherent instability of active vitamin C (L-ascorbic acid), however, remains the major therapeutic challenge. When exposed to air, L-ascorbic acid converts to inactive brown dihydroascorbic acid. To overcome the problem of instability, vitamin C and vitamin E preparations have been stabilized with ferulic acid. Ferulic acid is a potent antioxidant present in the cell walls of grains, fruits, and vegetables. The acid itself absorbs UV radiation, acting as a sunscreen. When mixed with vitamins E and C, it stabilizes the formulation and doubles synergistic photoprotection from fourfold (combined vitamins C and E) to eightfold (vitamin C, vitamin E, ferulic acid; C E ferulic).[80] Clinical studies show that topical C E ferulic acid provides substantial protection for human skin against solar simulator-induced oxidative skin damage, including erythema, sunburn cell formation, and cancer related DNA mutations.[86]

Yquem

Yquem extract is a novel, highly potent antioxidant. In in vitro studies it has been shown to cause highly significant reduction of oxidative stress. The antioxidant power of yquem extract at low concentrations (1.5 µg/mL) is highly superior to that of vitamin C (at 50 µM) and that of vitamin E (at 25µM). In a clinical study of 10 subjects, the extract was applied for 1 day to facial skin, and the rates of free-radical production were measured 18 hours after the last application and compared with an untreated zone. Treatment with yquem extract decreased the rate of free-radical production by 22% compared with untreated control. By comparison, grape polyphenols and idebendone formulations decreased free-radical production by only 2.3% and 4.1%, respectively.[9]

Coffeeberry

Polyphenols including chlorogenic acid, quinic acid, ferulic acid, and condensed proanthocyanidins are the active ingredients in coffeeberry, the fruit of the coffee plant *Coffea arabica*.[87] The antioxidant properties of polyphenols are related to their ability to quench free radicals. In in vitro testing with the oxygen radical absorbance capacity (ORAC) assay, coffeeberry was superior to other commonly used antioxidants, such as green tea extract, pomegranate extract, vitamin C, and vitamin E.[81,88] The clinical relevance of in vitro ORAC testing is controversial, especially because the ORAC scale was originally developed to determine the antioxidant potential of ingested, rather than topically applied, antioxidants.[89]

In a 6-week double-blind clinical trial, 30 patients with significant actinic damage used a skin regimen of 0.1% to 1% coffeeberry in skin cleansers and facial creams (commercially available as the RevaléSkin line, Stiefel). Compared with pretreatment, all patients saw statistically significant improvements in fine lines, wrinkles, pigmentation, and overall skin appearance[88]

Idebenone

This is a low-molecular-weight synthetic analog of coenzyme Q10. Because of its lower molecular weight, idebenone can penetrate the skin more efficiently than coenzyme Q10. In a clinical study of 50 subjects with moderate photoaging, an application of 0.5% to 1% idebenone lotion twice daily for 6 weeks reduced fine lines and wrinkles by 26% and 27%, respectively. Both groups saw a 37% improvement in skin hydration and a 30% to 33% improvement in global photoaging.[90]

Vine shoot

A new generation of ultrapotent antioxidants include *Vitis vinifera* shoot, a polyphenol-rich antioxidant and ectoine/hydroine, a natural blend of compounds found in halophilic microorganisms growing in extreme temperature and salinity. In a clinical study, 56 subjects were treated with a combination of *Vitis vinifera* shoot extract (0.045%) and ectoine/hydroine (1%). The combination was applied for a 4-week period twice daily; 90% of patients experienced a 25% overall improvement (firmness, radiant glow, evenness, smoothness, hydration, texture, softness) as assessed by an independent investigator. In in vitro assays, the antioxidant capacity of *Vitis vinifera* shoot appeared to be significantly more powerful than that of vitamin C or E.[91]

Soy

Isoflavones, including genistein and diadzein, are the main active ingredients and chemoprotective agents derived from soy. Other biologically active ingredients include essential fatty acids and amino acids, phytosterols, and small protein serine protease inhibitors such as Bowman-Birk inhibitor (BBI) and soy trypsin inhibitor (STI). By inhibiting protease-activated receptor 2 (PAR-2), STI inhibits melanosome transfer to keratinocytes.[92] Clinically, soy provides gentle anti-inflammatory, photoprotective, and skin lightening properties. Daily, or twice daily, application of a topical soy formulation over a 12-week period resulted in improved overall skin tone and texture, hyperpigmentation, skin blotchiness, and dullness (Diane Berson, MD, personal communication, 2009). In a clinical study of 6 adult patients, genistein showed a dose-dependent inhibition of UBV-induced erythema.[93]

Sunscreens

Broad-spectrum UVA and UVB sunscreens are the cornerstone of photoaging therapy. UVR causes several acute effects in the skin, including photosynthesis of vitamin D, immediate pigment darkening, delayed tanning, sunburn, epidermal thickening, and numerous immunologic effects, from altered antigen presentation to release of immunosuppressive factors.

UVA and UVB radiation contribute to the disruption of the extracellular matrix, a hallmark of photoaging. The presence of dermal changes in the deep reticular dermis, however, suggests that UVA radiation plays a key role, because only a small percentage of UVB penetrates into the superficial papillary dermis.[94,95] The mechanism of UVR mediated dermal damage includes:

1. Decreased collagen I and III synthesis
2. Increased collagen degradation by transforming growth factor-β (TGF-β) and activator protein A
3. Infiltration of inflammatory cells, predominately neutrophils, into the dermis
4. Release of ROS from neutrophils

Benzophenones (dioxybenzone, oxybenzone, sulisobenzone) provide protection in the UVB and UVA II range (320–340 nm). Currently, only oxybenzone is approved for use in the United States.

Avobenzone (Parson 1789), a dibenzoylmethane, absorbs in the UVA I (340–400 nm) range. However, its use is limited by its relative instability. Estimates suggest that all avobenzone is inactivated after 5 hours of sun exposure, equivalent to 50 J of solar energy. Stability of the avobenzone is markedly increased by combining with oxybenzone and 2,6-diethylhexylnaphthalate in commercially available Helioplex (Neutrogena). Another agent offering long-lasting short-wave UVA protection and photostabilization of avobenzone is ecamsule, commercially available as Mexoryl (L'Oreal, France).

Retinoids

The biologic properties of retinoids include free-radical scavenging and antioxidant activity, increasing fibroblast proliferation, modulation of cellular proliferation and differentiation, increased collagen and hyaluronate synthesis, and decreased matrix metalloproteinase mediated extracellular matrix degradation. Retinoids are therefore ideal for the treatment of photoaging.[96] Numerous studies have confirmed the clinical efficacy of various retinoids.[27,96–101] Histologic responses to chronic topical retinoid application include hyperproliferation, leading to a dose-dependent expansion of the numbers of cell layers of stratum spinosum and stratum granulosum, and elongation of the basal layer keratinocytes.

Chemical Peels

The efficacy of chemical peels for the treatment of photodamage has been widely reported.[102,103] Histologically, different chemical peels, GA, SA and LHA, alter the epidermis toward a non–sun-damaged pattern with keratinocytes showing a return of polarity, and more regular distribution of melanocytes and melanin granules.

In a randomized, right/left split-face controlled clinical trial of 43 women aged 35 to 60 years with fine lines, wrinkles, and dyschromia, application of 4 LHA (5%–10%) treatments was equivalent to 6 treatment sessions with GA (20%–50%). Both chemical peels were well tolerated and showed a significant reduction of all study parameters (fine lines, wrinkles, and hyperpigmentation) (LaRoche Posay, 2008, clinical data on file).

Laser Skin Resurfacing

The carbon dioxide and Er:YAG lasers remain gold standard for rejuvenation of photoaged skin. However, their use is associated with a risk of side effects and a prolonged postoperative recovery period. Newer rejuvenating laser systems offer the benefit of stimulation of collagen production and remodeling with little or no healing time and decreased patient discomfort.

Nonablative laser systems currently available include:

1. Mid-IR lasers targeting the dermis (Nd:YAG [1320 nm], diode [1450 μm])
2. Visible lasers, such as the PDL (585-595 nm) the pulsed KTP (532 nm) and Nd:YAG (1064 nm)
3. IPL
4. A combination of electrical (radiofrequency) and optical devices

Fractional resurfacing offers partial benefits of the ablative laser with faster recovery and fewer side effects. In addition to the original Fraxel SR (1550 nm erbium, Reliant Technologies), the Fraxel SR1500, Fraxel AFR (both Reliant Technologies), Lux 1540 Fractional (1540 nm, Palomar Medical Technologies, Burlington, Massachusetts), and Affirm (1320 nm plus 1440 nm, Cynosure Inc., Westford, Massachusetts) have been developed.[104]

COLLAGEN REPAIR
Introduction

The use of signaling peptides, growth factors (GF) and cytokines in collagen repair and clinical rejuvenation has emerged as an exciting new antiaging treatment option. Advances in basic research into wound healing, with the identification of key wound healing mediators, prompted translational clinical research on repair and remodeling of dermal infrastructure. The GFs implicated in wound healing are listed in **Table 1**.

GFs

Cell rejuvenation serum (CRS, Topix Pharmaceuticals, New York) relies on liposomal technology for dermal delivery of TGF-β1, L-ascorbic acid, and black cohosh (*Cimicifuga racemosa*). In a split-face clinical study of 12 patients with moderate facial photoaging, patients applied CRS cream with TGF-β1 to one side of the face and CRS cream without TGF-β1 to the opposite side. The results showed a statistically significant improvement of facial rhytids with the CRS cream containing TGF-β1 compared with the L-ascorbic acid and black cohosh only CRS preparation.[105]

NouriCel-MD, a proprietary mix of GFs, cytokines, and soluble proteins secreted by cultured neonatal human dermal fibroblasts during production of extracellular matrix in an oil-free gel, is currently available as TNS Recovery Complex (SkinMedica Inc., Carlsbad, California). In a clinical study, 14 patients with marked photodamage applied TNS Recovery Complex twice daily to facial skin for 60 days. The results showed a 15% to 35% decrease in fine lines and wrinkles as assessed by optical profilometry assay. In addition, thickening of the Grenz zone, new collagen formation (average 36%) and epidermal thickening (average 30%) were noted.[106]

The main ingredients in Bio-Restorative Skin Cream (Neocutis, Inc., San Francisco, CA) are processed skin-cell proteins, a proprietary blend of GFs, and cytokines extracted from cultured first trimester fetal human dermal fibroblasts. Compared with adult fibroblasts, fetal fibroblasts express only transient and low amounts of TGF-β1, which may contribute to virtually scarless healing in the first trimester of pregnancy.[107] Clinical benefits of Bio-Restorative Skin Cream were studied in 18 patients with moderate to severe photodamage. Twice daily application of Bio-Restorative Skin Cream for 60 days resulted in a 17% and 13% decrease in periorbital and perioral rhytids. Improvements in skin texture were also noted.[108]

Peptides

Cosmeceutical peptides, short-chain sequences of amino acids, are a rapidly expanding category of cosmeceuticals. Biologic effects of peptides may relate to their ability to enhance collagen production, relax dynamic skin wrinkling, and improve skin hydration and barrier function. The three main classes of peptides are signal peptides, neuropeptides, and carrier peptides.

Signal peptides
Signal peptides increase fibroblast production of collagen or decrease collagenase breakdown of existing collagen. Examples of signal peptides include valine-glycine-alanine-proline-glycine

Table 1
GF and cytokine signals involved in wound healing

GF	Cell Target and Effect
Heparin-binding epidermal growth factor-like growth factor (HB-EGF)	Keratinocyte and fibroblast mitogen
Fibroblastic growth factor (FGF) 1, 2, 4	Angiogenic, fibroblast mitogen
Platelet-derived growth factor (PDGF)	Chemotaxis of macrophages and fibroblasts; macrophage activation; fibroblasts mitogen, matrix production
Insulin-like growth factor 1 (IGF-1)	Endothelial cells and fibroblast mitogen
TGF-β1 and β2	Keratinocyte migration; chemotaxis for macrophages and fibroblast
TGF-β3	Antiscarring
IL-1α and -β	Early activators of GF expression in macrophages, keratinocytes and fibroblasts
TNF α	Mechanism of action similar to IL-1α and -β

Data from Mehta RC, Fitzpatrick RE. Endogenous growth factors as cosmeceuticals. Dermatol Ther 2007;20(5):350–9.

peptide,[109,110] lysine-threonine-threonine-lysine-serine peptide (KTTKS),[111] tyrosine-tyrosine-arginine-alanine-aspartame-aspartame-alanine peptide, and glycyl-L-histadyl-L-lysine (GHK) peptide.

Application of elastin-derived valine-glycine-alanine-proline-glycine peptide has been shown to significantly stimulate human dermal skin fibroblast production and down-regulate elastin expression. Palmitate-bound valine-glycine-alanine-proline-glycine peptide is commercially available in a number of cosmetic preparations under the trade name of palmitoyl oligopeptide.[2]

Palmitate-bound KTTKS peptide (pal-KTTKS, palmitoyl pentapeptide-3, trade name Matrixyl, Sederma, France) is a fragment of type I procollagen. Of the many collagen breakdown products, pentapeptide KTTKS was shown to have the highest fibroblast stimulation properties in in vitro subconfluent monolayer cultures. Exposure of fibroblasts to collagen degradation products is hypothesized to induce cellular collagen repair with enhanced collagen synthesis and down-regulation of matrix collagenases. Pentapeptide was shown to stimulate new collagen synthesis and increase production of extracellular matrix proteins such as type I and II collagen and fibronectin.[112] Matrixyl contains 800 parts per million of pal-KTTKS, and currently available cosmetic preparations contain 1 to 4 parts per million of pal-KTTKS.[6] In a 12-week double-blind, placebo-controlled, split-face study of 93 Caucasian women, pal-KTTKS provided significant improvement of wrinkles and fine lines compared with the placebo group by qualitative technical and expert grader image analysis.[113]

Neuropeptides

Also known as neurotransmitter-affecting peptides, neuropeptides mimic the effects of botulinum neurotoxin. Clinically, neuropeptides decrease facial muscle contraction, reducing lines and wrinkles by raising the threshold for minimal muscle activity. Over time, they are postulated to also reduce subconscious muscle movement. The properties of several neuropeptides are discussed below. For a comprehensive review see Lupo and colleagues.[2]

Neuropeptides are designed to block individual components of the neuromuscular junction (NMJ). Most neuropeptides act on the soluble N-ethylmaleimide-sensitive factor attachment protein receptors (SNARE) complex, a component of the NMJ. Whether topically applied neuropeptides can truly penetrate to the level of the NMJ remains to be tested.

Acetyl-hexapeptide-3 (AC-gly glu-met-gln-arg-arg-NH$_2$) is a synthetic peptide patterned after the N-terminus of SNAP-25, an inhibitor of SNARE complex formation and catecholamine release. This peptide is currently marketed as Argireline (McEit International Trade Co., Ltd.).[114] In one open-label trial, 10 female patients applied a 5% acetyl-hexapeptide-3 cream twice daily. Subjects experienced a 27% improvement in periorbital rhytids after 30 days as measured by silica replica analysis.[114]

Pentapetide-3 (amino acid sequence not published), currently marketed as Vialox (Cellular Skin, Rx) has a mechanism of action similar to that of tubocurarine, the main ingredient of curare. Its mechanism of action is competitive inhibition of acetylcholine postsynaptic membrane receptor. Acetylcholine receptor blockage in turn prevents muscle contraction.[2]

Carrier peptides

Carrier peptides stabilize and deliver trace elements necessary for wound healing, enzymatic processes, and collagen regeneration into the skin. The most commonly encountered carrier peptides stabilize and deliver copper, an elemental metal for proper wound healing, enzymatic processes (collagen and elastin synthesis, cytochrome c oxidase, down-regulation of MMPs and inhibition of collagenase), and cutaneous aniogenesis.[2] The copper peptide technology is currently adapted for anti-aging and general skin care in several skin care preparations. The tripeptide complex, GHK spontaneously complexes with copper and facilities its cellular uptake.[115] In vitro GHK-copper complex increases levels of tissue inhibitors of MMPs, stimulates collagen I and glycosoaminoglycans synthesis, and enzymatic actions of cytochrome c oxidase and tyrosinase.[116] Clinically, GHK-copper application led to an improvement in the appearance of fine lines/wrinkles and an increase in skin density and skin thickeness.[2]

Nonablative, Fractional and Ablative Laser Resurfacing

Cosmeceuticals directed at collagen repair may prove to be of pivotal importance when combined with nonablative, fractional, and ablative laser resurfacing. Laser resurfacing rejuvenates skin by producing controlled zones of dermal or epidermal wounding (epidermal damage is not seen with nonablative technologies). Subsequent inflammation and cytokine mediated superficial dermal healing and remodeling leads to clinical improvement. Application of GFs and collagen repair peptides might further accelerate or improve the wound healing process. Fractional and ablative, compared with nonablative, resurfacing provides an additional benefit of altering the barrier properties of the epidermis and may allow for enhanced penetration of GF and peptides in the immediate postoperative period. That, in theory, may offer deeper penetration and pandermal rejuvenation. Preprocedural treatment with GF and peptides may prime the skin, allowing for a more robust rejuvenating response to laser resurfacing.

REFERENCES

1. Kligman A. The future of cosmeceuticals: an interview with Albert Kligman, MD, PhD. Interview by Zoe Diana Draelos. Dermatol Surg 2005;31(7 Pt 2):890–1.
2. Lupo MP, Cole AL. Cosmeceutical peptides. Dermatol Ther 2007;20(5):343–9.
3. Choi CM, Berson DS. Cosmeceuticals. Semin Cutan Med Surg 2006;25(3):163–8.
4. Berson DS. Natural antioxidants. J Drugs Dermatol 2008;7(7 Suppl):s7–12.
5. Draelos ZD. Skin lightening preparations and the hydroquinone controversy. Dermatol Ther 2007; 20(5):308–13.
6. Draelos ZD. The cosmeceutical realm. Clin Dermatol 2008;26(6):627–32.
7. Draelos ZD. Topical agents used in association with cosmetic surgery. Semin Cutan Med Surg 1999; 18(2):112–8.
8. Lawrence N, Bligard CA, Reed R, et al. Exogenous ochronosis in the United States. J Am Acad Dermatol 1988;18(5 Pt 2):1207–11.
9. Westerhof W, Kooyers TJ. Hydroquinone and its analogues in dermatology – a potential health risk. J Cosmet Dermatol 2005;4(2):55–9.
10. Fitton A, Goa KL. Azelaic acid. A review of its pharmacological properties and therapeutic efficacy in acne and hyperpigmentary skin disorders. Drugs 1991;41(5):780–98.
11. Balina LM, Graupe K. The treatment of melasma. 20% azelaic acid versus 4% hydroquinone cream. Int J Dermatol 1991;30(12):893–5.
12. Bissett D. Topical niacinamide and barrier enhancement. Cutis 2002;70(6 Suppl):8–12.
13. Bissett DL, Oblong JE, Berge CA. Niacinamide: A B vitamin that improves aging facial skin appearance. Dermatol Surg 2005;31(7 Pt 2): 860–5.
14. Greatens A, Hakozaki T, Koshoffer A, et al. Effective inhibition of melanosome transfer to keratinocytes by lectins and niacinamide is reversible. Exp Dermatol 2005;14(7):498–508.
15. Bissett DL, Robinson LR, Raleigh PS, et al. Reduction in the appearance of facial hyperpigmentation by topical N-acetyl glucosamine. J Cosmet Dermatol 2007;6(1):20–6.
16. Amer M, Metwalli M. Topical liquiritin improves melasma. Int J Dermatol 2000;39(4):299–301.
17. Yokota T, Nishio H, Kubota Y, et al. The inhibitory effect of glabridin from licorice extracts on melanogenesis and inflammation. Pigment Cell Res 1998; 11(6):355–61.
18. Hori I, Nihei K, Kubo I. Structural criteria for depigmenting mechanism of arbutin. Phytother Res 2004;18(6):475–9.
19. Hamed SH, Sriwiriyanont P, deLong MA, et al. Comparative efficacy and safety of deoxyarbutin, a new tyrosinase-inhibiting agent. J Cosmet Sci 2006;57(4):291–308.
20. Choi S, Lee SK, Kim JE, et al. Aloesin inhibits hyperpigmentation induced by UV radiation. Clin Exp Dermatol 2002;27(6):513–5.

21. Jones K, Hughes J, Hong M, et al. Modulation of melanogenesis by aloesin: a competitive inhibitor of tyrosinase. Pigment Cell Res 2002;15(5): 335–40.

22. Wang Z, Li X, Yang Z, et al. Effects of aloesin on melanogenesis in pigmented skin equivalents. Int J Cosmet Sci 2008;30(2):121–30.

23. Lazou K, Sadick NS, Kurfurst R, et al. The use of antisense strategy to modulate human melanogenesis. J Drugs Dermatol 2007;6(6 Suppl):s2–7.

24. Lee GS. Intravenous vitamin C in the treatment of post-laser hyperpigmentation for melasma: a short report. J Cosmet Laser Ther 2008;10(4): 234–6.

25. Soliman MM, Ramadan SA, Bassiouny DA, et al. Combined trichloroacetic acid peel and topical ascorbic acid versus trichloroacetic acid peel alone in the treatment of melasma: a comparative study. J Cosmet Dermatol 2007;6(2):89–94.

26. Espinal-Perez LE, Moncada B, Castanedo-Cazares JP. A double-blind randomized trial of 5% ascorbic acid vs. 4% hydroquinone in melasma. Int J Dermatol 2004;43(8):604–7.

27. Kaidbey KH, Kligman AM, Yoshida H. Effects of intensive application of retinoic acid on human skin. Br J Dermatol 1975;92(6):693–701.

28. Kligman AM, Willis I. A new formula for depigmenting human skin. Arch Dermatol 1975;111(1):40–8.

29. Gupta AK, Gover MD, Nouri K, et al. The treatment of melasma: a review of clinical trials. J Am Acad Dermatol 2006;55(6):1048–65.

30. Griffiths CE, Finkel LJ, Ditre CM, et al. Topical tretinoin (retinoic acid) improves melasma. A vehicle-controlled, clinical trial. Br J Dermatol 1993;129(4):415–21.

31. Rahman Z, Alam M, Dover JS. Fractional laser treatment for pigmentation and texture improvement. Skin Therapy Lett 2006;11(9):7–11.

32. Goldberg DJ, Berlin AL, Phelps R. Histologic and ultrastructural analysis of melasma after fractional resurfacing. Lasers Surg Med 2008;40(2):134–8.

33. Tannous ZS, Astner S. Utilizing fractional resurfacing in the treatment of therapy-resistant melasma. J Cosmet Laser Ther 2005;7(1):39–43.

34. Rokhsar CK, Fitzpatrick RE. The treatment of melasma with fractional photothermolysis: a pilot study. Dermatol Surg 2005;31(12):1645–50.

35. Kunachak S, Leelaudomlipi P, Wongwaisayawan S. Dermabrasion: a curative treatment for melasma. Aesthetic Plast Surg 2001;25(2):114–7.

36. Grimes PE. The safety and efficacy of salicylic acid chemical peels in darker racial-ethnic groups. Dermatol Surg 1999;25(1):18–22.

37. Erbil H, Sezer E, Tastan B, et al. Efficacy and safety of serial glycolic acid peels and a topical regimen in the treatment of recalcitrant melasma. J Dermatol 2007;34(1):25–30.

38. Lim JT, Tham SN. Glycolic acid peels in the treatment of melasma among Asian women. Dermatol Surg 1997;23(3):177–9.

39. Reszko AE, Granstein. Pathogenesis of rosacea. J Cosmet Dermatol 2008;21(4):224–32.

40. Weber TM, Ceilley RI, Buerger A, et al. Skin tolerance, efficacy, and quality of life of patients with red facial skin using a skin care regimen containing Licochalcone A. J Cosmet Dermatol 2006;5(3): 227–32.

41. Kolbe L, Immeyer J, Batzer J, et al. Anti-inflammatory efficacy of Licochalcone A: correlation of clinical potency and in vitro effects. Arch Dermatol Res 2006;298(1):23–30.

42. Del Rosso JQ. The use of topical azelaic acid for common skin disorders other than inflammatory rosacea. Cutis 2006;77(2 Suppl):22–4.

43. Bedi MK, Shenefelt PD. Herbal therapy in dermatology. Arch Dermatol 2002;138(2):232–42.

44. Syed TA, Ahmad SA, Holt AH, et al. Management of psoriasis with aloe vera extract in a hydrophilic cream: a placebo-controlled, double-blind study. Trop Med Int Health 1996;1(4):505–9.

45. Brown DJ, Dattner AM. Phytotherapeutic approaches to common dermatologic conditions. Arch Dermatol 1998;134(11):1401–4.

46. Albring M, Albrecht H, Alcorn G, et al. The measuring of the antiinflammatory effect of a compound on the skin of volunteers. Methods Find Exp Clin Pharmacol 1983;5(8):575–7.

47. Wu J. Anti-inflammatory ingredients. J Drugs Dermatol 2008;7(7 Suppl):s13–6.

48. Martin K, Sur R, Liebel F, et al. Parthenolide-depleted feverfew (Tanacetum parthenium) protects skin from UV irradiation and external aggression. Arch Dermatol Res 2008;300(2): 69–80.

49. FDA, Department of Health and Human Services [HHS]. Skin protectant drug products for over-the-counter human use; final monograph. Final rule. Fed Regist 2003;68(33):362–81.

50. Kurtz ES, Wallo W. Colloidal oatmeal: history, chemistry and clinical properties. J Drugs Dermatol 2007;6(2):167–70.

51. Torras MA, Faura CA, Schonlau F, et al. Antimicrobial activity of Pycnogenol. Phytother Res 2005; 19(7):647–8.

52. Sime S, Reeve VE. Protection from inflammation, immunosuppression and carcinogenesis induced by UV radiation in mice by topical Pycnogenol. Photochem Photobiol 2004;79(2):193–8.

53. Rohdewald P. A review of the French maritime pine bark extract (Pycnogenol), a herbal medication with a diverse clinical pharmacology. Int J Clin Pharmacol Ther 2002;40(4):158–68.

54. Saliou C, Rimbach G, Moini H, et al. Solar ultraviolet-induced erythema in human skin and nuclear

factor-kappa-B-dependent gene expression in keratinocytes are modulated by a French maritime pine bark extract. Free Radic Biol Med 2001; 30(2):154–60.

55. Andreassi M, Stanghellini E, Ettorre A, et al. Antioxidant activity of topically applied lycopene. J Eur Acad Dermatol Venereol 2004;18(1):52–5.

56. Offord EA, Gautier JC, Avanti O, et al. Photoprotective potential of lycopene, beta-carotene, vitamin E, vitamin C and carnosic acid in UVA-irradiated human skin fibroblasts. Free Radic Biol Med 2002;32(12):1293–303.

57. Pinnell SR. Cutaneous photodamage, oxidative stress, and topical antioxidant protection. J Am Acad Dermatol 2003;48(1):1–19.

58. Singh RP, Agarwal R. Flavonoid antioxidant silymarin and skin cancer. Antioxid Redox Signal 2002; 4(4):655–63.

59. Katiyar SK, Roy AM, Baliga MS. Silymarin induces apoptosis primarily through a p53-dependent pathway involving Bcl-2/Bax, cytochrome c release, and caspase activation. Mol Cancer Ther 2005;4(2):207–16.

60. Katiyar SK. Silymarin and skin cancer prevention: anti-inflammatory, antioxidant and immunomodulatory effects [review]. Int J Oncol 2005;26(1): 169–76.

61. Berardesca E, Cameli N, Cavallotti C, et al. Combined effects of silymarin and methylsulfonylmethane in the management of rosacea: clinical and instrumental evaluation. J Cosmet Dermatol 2008;7(1):8–14.

62. Erden IM, Kahraman A, Koken T. Beneficial effects of quercetin on oxidative stress induced by ultraviolet A. Clin Exp Dermatol 2001;26(6):536–9.

63. Piantelli M, Maggiano N, Ricci R, et al. Tamoxifen and quercetin interact with type II estrogen binding sites and inhibit the growth of human melanoma cells. J Invest Dermatol 1995;105(2):248–53.

64. Thornfeldt C. Cosmeceuticals containing herbs: fact, fiction, and future. Dermatol Surg 2005; 31(7 Pt 2):873–80.

65. Taub AF. Procedural treatments for acne vulgaris. Dermatol Surg 2007;33(9):1005–26.

66. Kessler E, Flanagan K, Chia C, et al. Comparison of alpha- and beta-hydroxy acid chemical peels in the treatment of mild to moderately severe facial acne vulgaris. Dermatol Surg 2008;34(1):45–50.

67. Lee HS, Kim IH. Salicylic acid peels for the treatment of acne vulgaris in Asian patients. Dermatol Surg 2003;29(12):1196–9.

68. Corcuff P, Fiat F, Minondo AM, et al. A comparative ultrastructural study of hydroxyacids induced desquamation. Eur J Dermatol 2002;12(4). XXXIX–XLIII.

69. Uhoda E, Pierard-Franchimont C, Pierard GE. Comedolysis by a lipohydroxyacid formulation in acne-prone subjects. Eur J Dermatol 2003;13(1): 65–8.

70. Lowe NJ, Behr KL, Fitzpatrick R, et al. Flash lamp pumped dye laser for rosacea-associated telangiectasia and erythema. J Dermatol Surg Oncol 1991;17(6):522–5.

71. Butterwick KJ, Butterwick LS, Han A. Laser and light therapies for acne rosacea. J Drugs Dermatol 2006;5(1):35–9.

72. Yamasaki K, Di NA, Bardan A, et al. Increased serine protease activity and cathelicidin promotes skin inflammation in rosacea. Nat Med 2007; 13(8):975–80.

73. Barak O, Treat JR, James WD. Antimicrobial peptides: effectors of innate immunity in the skin. Adv Dermatol 2005;21:357–74.

74. Harvey J. Rosacea: molecular insights. Skin Aging 2007;14.

75. Kosmadaki MG, Gilchrest BA. The role of telomeres in skin aging/photoaging. Micron 2004;35(3): 155–9.

76. Gilchrest BA. Skin aging and photoaging: an overview. J Am Acad Dermatol 1989;21(3 Pt 2): 610–3.

77. Schwartz E, Cruickshank FA, Christensen CC, et al. Collagen alterations in chronically sun-damaged human skin. Photochem Photobiol 1993;58(6): 841–4.

78. Camouse MM, Hanneman KK, Conrad EP, et al. Protective effects of tea polyphenols and caffeine. Expert Rev Anticancer Ther 2005;5(6):1061–8.

79. Katiyar SK, Elmets CA, Agarwal R, et al. Protection against ultraviolet-B radiation-induced local and systemic suppression of contact hypersensitivity and edema responses in C3H/HeN mice by green tea polyphenols. Photochem Photobiol 1995;62(5): 855–61.

80. Wang ZY, Agarwal R, Bickers DR, et al. Protection against ultraviolet B radiation-induced photocarcinogenesis in hairless mice by green tea polyphenols. Carcinogenesis 1991;12(8):1527–30.

81. Vayalil PK, Mittal A, Hara Y, et al. Green tea polyphenols prevent ultraviolet light-induced oxidative damage and matrix metalloproteinases expression in mouse skin. J Invest Dermatol 2004;122(6): 1480–7.

82. Katiyar SK, Afaq F, Perez A, et al. Green tea polyphenol (−)-epigallocatechin-3-gallate treatment of human skin inhibits ultraviolet radiation-induced oxidative stress. Carcinogenesis 2001;22(2): 287–94.

83. Elmets CA, Singh D, Tubesing K, et al. Cutaneous photoprotection from ultraviolet injury by green tea polyphenols. J Am Acad Dermatol 2001;44(3): 425–32.

84. Chiu AE, Chan JL, Kern DG, et al. Double-blinded, placebo-controlled trial of green tea extracts in the

clinical and histologic appearance of photoaging skin. Dermatol Surg 2005;31(7 Pt 2):855–60.

85. Fitzpatrick RE, Rostan EF. Double-blind, half-face study comparing topical vitamin C and vehicle for rejuvenation of photodamage. Dermatol Surg 2002;28(3):231–6.

86. Lin FH, Lin JY, Gupta RD, et al. Ferulic acid stabilizes a solution of vitamins C and E and doubles its photoprotection of skin. J Invest Dermatol 2005;125(4):826–32.

87. Baumann LS. Less-known botanical cosmeceuticals. Dermatol Ther 2007;20(5):330–42.

88. Farris P. Idebenone, green tea, and coffeeberry extract: new and innovative antioxidants. Dermatol Ther 2007;20(5):322–9.

89. Ditre C, Wu J, Baumann LS, et al. Innovations in natural antioxidants and their role in dermatology. Cutis 2008;82(6 Suppl):2–16.

90. McDaniel D, Neudecker B, Dinardo J, et al. Clinical efficacy assessment in photodamaged skin of 0.5% and 1.0% idebenone. J Cosmet Dermatol 2005;4(3):167–73.

91. Cornacchione S, Sadick NS, Neveu M, et al. In vivo skin antioxidant effect of a new combination based on a specific *Vitis vinifera* shoot extract and a biotechnological extract. J Drugs Dermatol 2007;6(6 Suppl):s8–13.

92. Seiberg M, Paine C, Sharlow E, et al. The protease-activated receptor 2 regulates pigmentation via keratinocyte-melanocyte interactions. Exp Cell Res 2000;254(1):25–32.

93. Wei H, Saladi R, Lu Y, et al. Isoflavone genistein: photoprotection and clinical implications in dermatology. J Nutr 2003;133(11 Suppl 1):3811S–9S.

94. Lim HH, Buttery JE. Determination of ethanol in serum by an enzymatic PMS-INT colorimetric method. Clin Chim Acta 1977;75(1):9–12.

95. Talwar HS, Griffiths CE, Fisher GJ, et al. Reduced type I and type III procollagens in photodamaged adult human skin. J Invest Dermatol 1995;105(2):285–90.

96. Sorg O, Kuenzli S, Kaya G, et al. Proposed mechanisms of action for retinoid derivatives in the treatment of skin aging. J Cosmet Dermatol 2005;4(4):237–44.

97. Stefanaki C, Stratigos A, Katsambas A. Topical retinoids in the treatment of photoaging. J Cosmet Dermatol 2005;4(2):130–4.

98. Singh M, Griffiths CE. The use of retinoids in the treatment of photoaging. Dermatol Ther 2006;19(5):297–305.

99. Serri R, Iorizzo M. Cosmeceuticals: focus on topical retinoids in photoaging. Clin Dermatol 2008;26(6):633–5.

100. Mukherjee S, Date A, Patravale V, et al. Retinoids in the treatment of skin aging: an overview of clinical efficacy and safety. Clin Interv Aging 2006;1(4):327–48.

101. Helfrich YR, Sachs DL, Voorhees JJ. Overview of skin aging and photoaging. Dermatol Nurs 2008;20(3):177–83.

102. Monheit GD, Chastain MA. Chemical peels. Facial Plast Surg Clin North Am 2001;9(2):239–55, viii.

103. Clark E, Scerri L. Superficial and medium-depth chemical peels. Clin Dermatol 2008;26(2):209–18.

104. Alexiades-Armenakas MR, Dover JS, Arndt KA. The spectrum of laser skin resurfacing: nonablative, fractional, and ablative laser resurfacing. J Am Acad Dermatol 2008;58(5):719–37.

105. Ehrlich M, Rao J, Pabby A, et al. Improvement in the appearance of wrinkles with topical transforming growth factor beta(1) and l-ascorbic acid. Dermatol Surg 2006;32(5):618–25.

106. Fitzpatrick RE, Rostan EF. Reversal of photodamage with topical growth factors: a pilot study. J Cosmet Laser Ther 2003;5(1):25–34.

107. Cass DL, Meuli M, Adzick NS. Scar wars: implications of fetal wound healing for the pediatric burn patient. Pediatr Surg Int 1997;12(7):484–9.

108. Gold MH, Goldman MP, Biron J. Efficacy of novel skin cream containing mixture of human growth factors and cytokines for skin rejuvenation. J Drugs Dermatol 2007;6(2):197–201.

109. Tajima S, Wachi H, Uemura Y, et al. Modulation by elastin peptide VGVAPG of cell proliferation and elastin expression in human skin fibroblasts. Arch Dermatol Res 1997;289(8):489–92.

110. Kamoun A, Landeau JM, Godeau G, et al. Growth stimulation of human skin fibroblasts by elastin-derived peptides. Cell Adhes Commun 1995;3(4):273–81.

111. Lintner K. Promoting production in the extracellular matrix without compromising barrier. Cutis 2002;70(6 Suppl):13–6.

112. Katayama K, Armendariz-Borunda J, Raghow R, et al. A pentapeptide from type I procollagen promotes extracellular matrix production. J Biol Chem 1993;268(14):9941–4.

113. Robinson LR, Fitzgerald NC, Doughty DG, et al. Topical palmitoyl pentapeptide provides improvement in photoaged human facial skin. Int J Cosmet Sci 2005;27(3):155–60.

114. Blanes-Mira C, Clemente J, Jodas G, et al. A synthetic hexapeptide (Argireline) with antiwrinkle activity. Int J Cosmet Sci 2002;24(5):303–10.

115. Pickart L, Freedman JH, Loker WJ, et al. Growth-modulating plasma tripeptide may function by facilitating copper uptake into cells. Nature 1980;288(5792):715–7.

116. Buffoni F, Pino R, Dal PA. Effect of tripeptide-copper complexes on the process of skin wound healing and on cultured fibroblasts. Arch Int Pharmacodyn Ther 1995;330(3):345–60.

Botulinum Toxin in Facial Rejuvenation: An Update

Jean Carruthers, MD[a],*, Alastair Carruthers, MD[b]

KEYWORDS
- Botox • Rejuvenation • Facial reshaping
- Adjunctive uses • Safety • Predictability

Since its initial approval by the US Food and Drug Administration (FDA) 20 years ago for the treatment of strabismus, hemifacial spasm, and blepharospasm in adults, botulinum toxin (BTX) has become one of the most frequently requested products in cosmetic rejuvenation around the world. After years of clinical success and consistent safety in the upper face, the use of BTX has expanded and evolved to include increasingly complicated indications. In the hands of adept injectors, the focus has shifted from the treatment of individual dynamic rhytides to shaping, contouring, and sculpting, alone or in combination with other cosmetic procedures, to enhance the aesthetic appearance of the face. Although recent reports have questioned the safety of BTX, 25 years of therapeutic and over 20 years of cosmetic use has demonstrated an impressive record of safety and efficacy when used appropriately by experienced injectors.

HISTORY AND CLINICAL DEVELOPMENT

First identified well over 100 years ago as a cause of food poisoning, the bacterium *Clostridium botulinum* was studied extensively over the next 50 years, leading to the identification of seven distinct serotypes, and the isolation and purification of BTX type A (BTX-A).[1,2] In 1980s, Scott published the landmark paper establishing the safety of BTX-A in humans for the treatment of strabismus.[3] In 1987, Carruthers and Carruthers noticed that patients treated for blepharospasm also experienced an improvement in glabellar rhytides; the subsequent publication of their results[4] sparked a flurry of interest and additional studies.[5,6] Since then, BTX-A has been approved by the FDA for a variety of applications, including strabismus, blepharospasm, cervical dystonia, hyperhidrosis, and mild-to-moderate glabellar rhytides, and by Health Canada for facial wrinkling.

FORMULATIONS

The majority of peer-reviewed reports in the literature focus on the original formulation of BTX-A: BOTOX Cosmetic (Vistabel in most of Europe and Vistabex in Italy; Allergan, Inc., Irvine, California). BOTOX has been approved for 20 indications in more than 75 countries.[7] However, several other products are or will be available in the near future. Reloxin (Dysport; Ipsen Ltd., United Kingdom/Medicis, Scottsdale, Arizona) is expected to receive FDA approval for cosmetic applications in North America in April 2009 and has already received approval in 15 European countries as Azzalure (Galderma, France). Its UK counterpart, Dysport, is approved in over 65 countries for therapeutic indications and differs from BOTOX in purification procedures.[8] There is some evidence that Dysport may show greater diffusion and migration, with increased potential for side effects and less precise localization of clinical effects.[9–11] Dose ratios between Dysport and BOTOX have

[a] Department of Ophthalmology and Visual Sciences, University of British Columbia, 943 West Broadway, Suite 740, Vancouver, BC, Canada V5Z 4E1
[b] Department of Dermatology and Skin Science, University of British Columbia, 943 West Broadway, Suite 820, Vancoucer, BC, Canada V5Z 4E1
* Corresponding author.
E-mail address: drjean@carruthers.net (J. Carruthers).

Dermatol Clin 27 (2009) 417–425
doi:10.1016/j.det.2009.08.001
0733-8635/09/$ – see front matter © 2009 Published by Elsevier Inc.

ranged in the literature from 6:1 to 1:1, though new evidence suggests a more suitable dose ratio of less than 3:1.[12,13]

Xeomin (NT-201; Merz Pharmaceuticals, Frankfurt, Germany) is the third BTX-A licensed in Germany. It has received approval for the treatment of blepharospasm and cervical dystonia in some European countries, Mexico, and Argentina; for glabellar rhytides in Argentina; and is in Phase 3 testing for glabellar lines in North America.[8] In potency, Xeomin appears to exhibit a 1:1 dose ratio when compared with BOTOX,[14] and therapeutic clinical studies have found similar levels of efficacy and safety.[15,16] Xeomin is free of complexing proteins, which some believe may result in purer formulations with greater efficacy and a reduced risk of sensitization and antibody formation.[16]

The only available BTX type B in North America and Europe, Myobloc/NeuroBloc (Solstice Neurosciences Inc./Eisai Co., Ltd.) is approved for the treatment of cervical dystonia.[8] Clinical data indicate that injections of Myobloc for cosmetic applications are more painful with a shorter duration of effect,[17,18] but are associated with a more rapid onset of action and a greater area of diffusion.[19]

PureTox (Mentor Corporation, Santa Barbara, California) is an uncomplexed type A neurotoxin, similar to Xeomin, in Phase 3 testing for glabellar rhytides, and in various stages of development for therapeutic indications in the United States. Globally, several other BTX products are under development.[8] Chinese BTX-A (CBTX-A; marketed as Prosigne in Brazil; Lanzhou Institute of Biological Products, China) is the only approved BTX-A in China, contains bovine gelatin protein, and appears to be slightly less effective than BOTOX.[20] CBTX-A must be distinguished from CNBTX-A (Nanfeng Medical Science and Technology Development Co., Ltd), which is neither licensed nor approved in any country and contains significantly higher levels of BTX, despite appearances to the contrary when it is sold by way of the Internet. The high levels of BTX may constitute a severe health risk for patients.[21] Neuronox (Medy-Tox Inc., South Korea) is widely used in Korea and Southeast Asia. Little has been published about Neuronox, although Stone and colleagues report that Neuronox and BOTOX produce equivalent responses in a murine model.[22]

COSMETIC APPLICATIONS OF BOTULINUM TOXIN-A

Since the initial FDA approval of BTX-A for therapeutic applications, practitioners have employed the neurotoxin to treat a variety of hyperkinetic facial lines, including crow's feet, horizontal forehead lines and glabellar rhytides in the upper face (**Figs. 1–3**) and folds and lines in the lower face (see **Fig. 3**; **Figs. 4–7**), with a high level of efficacy and patient satisfaction.[23–28] As injector and recipient confidence has grown, so too have the areas of application; now, BTX-A is used to sculpt the face and restore symmetry, and is a useful adjunct to other cosmetic applications and surgery.

Facial Sculpting

In the upper face, BTX-A is capable of lifting the brow and widening the eyes. Several reports noted that injections in the glabella resulted in central, medial, and lateral brow elevation,[29–31] which has been shown to be the result of partial inactivation and increased resting tone of the frontalis.[31] Similarly, small doses of BTX-A injected into the lower pretarsal orbicularis open the palpebral aperture at rest and at smile in individuals who desire a wider, rounder eye.[32,33] In the lower face, BTX injections into the masseter can alter the shape of the jawline and has been well documented in East Asian populations, with up to 50% reduction in muscle thickness and bulk.[34–37] More recently, the toxin has been shown to be beneficial in improving the aesthetic appearance of the face in non-Asian populations.[38,39] Liew and Dart investigated the use of BTX for aesthetic reshaping of the mandibular angle in a Western population compared with an East Asian control group.[38] While all patients achieved aesthetic improvement of the shape of their lower face, aesthetic improvement in Western patients was achieved with smaller

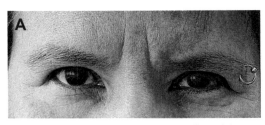
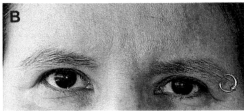

Fig. 1. Cosmetic use of BTX-A in the upper face: (*A*) prior to injection (*B*) and after treatment for glabellar lines, crow's feet, and horizontal forehead rhytides.

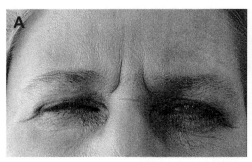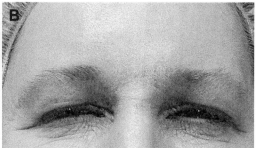

Fig. 2. Glabella before (*A*) and after (*B*) combined treatment with BTX-A and hyaluronic acid.

doses of BTX-A (25–30 U) compared to doses required in the East Asian control group (40 U), and the effects lasted for 9 to 12 months. Moreover, Western patients experienced additional improvement in function attributed to bruxism, an effect that has been noted elsewhere in the literature,[40] lasting for 6 to 7 months.

Adjunctive Botulinum Toxin-A

BTX-A is used increasingly in combination with other cosmetic procedures to prolong and enhance aesthetic results. The combination of BTX-A and soft-tissue augmentation is a highly synergistic approach used to achieve more effective, longer-lasting results by reducing the dynamic component of the target rhytide, especially when used in the glabella, brow, forehead, zygomatic and perioral regions, and in the neck.[41–44] Combination therapy leads to greater patients' satisfaction and superior efficacy compared with fillers alone (see **Fig. 3**).[43,45,46] Similarly, the benefits of laser resurfacing can be optimized by pretreatment with BTX-A, leading to superior and longer-lasting aesthetic outcomes.[42,47–49] Studies of Intense Pulsed Light show that combination therapy with BTX-A increases the overall aesthetic benefit and improves skin texture and the appearance of telangiectasias (see **Figs. 4** and **5**).[50,51]

Finally, many cosmetic surgeons consider BTX-A a key adjunct in surgical interventions; the neurotoxin serves to increase longevity of the procedure and aids in wound healing by reducing repetitive muscular actions that can hasten dehiscence.[42,47] Indeed, multiple trials have shown the benefit of BTX-A injections to facilitate wound healing; pretreating the underlying musculature with BTX-A allows for the use of finer sutures and minimizes scarring by reducing tension on the wound edge, allowing it to heal more readily (**Fig. 8**).[52–54]

SAFETY

Most side effects associated with the cosmetic application of BTX-A are mild and transient and include bruising, swelling, pain around the injection site, headache, and flu like symptoms.[55] More serious complications, such as brow or eyelid ptosis, can occur but are usually associated with poor injection technique and lack of injector experience and result from diffusion of the toxin into adjacent musculature.[56]

Clinical Safety Profile of Botulinum Toxin

Examination of nearly 20 years of research reveals an impressive record of safety and efficacy. Most reported adverse events (AE) are transient and mild. Coté and colleagues analyzed 995 cases of

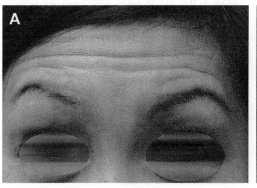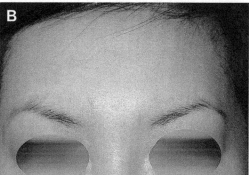

Fig. 3. Horizontal forehead lines before (*A*) and after (*B*) treatment with BTX-A.

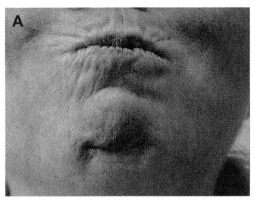
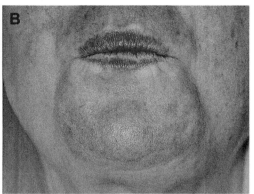

Fig. 4. Mental scar and mentalis muscle disinsertion before (A) and after (B) treatment with BTX-A.

nonserious side effects among 1031 AE reports submitted to the FDA; side effects included lack of intended cosmetic effect (63%), injection-site reaction (19%), ptosis (11%), muscle weakness (5%), and headache (5%).[57] Zagui and colleagues analyzed eight randomized trials and 13 case reports of cosmetic BTX up to September of 2007.[58] Of 1003 subjects, 182 (18.14%) experienced AE, of which eyelid ptosis was the most frequent (3.39%). Other side effects included headache, local reaction, and infection.

Long-term safety of multiple-injection sessions over time has been established by several analyses. Hsiung and colleagues examined 235 patients who received BTX-A injections for movement disorders over a 10-year period and found mostly minor AE in 27% of subjects.[59] Likewise, a review of 36 randomized trials and 1425 subjects who received BTX-A for therapeutic indications revealed no serious AE,[60] and the authors' own retrospective analysis of 853 upper-face treatment sessions in 50 subjects, for an average of 5.95 years, showed only 9 subjects reported AE, all transient and mild to moderate in severity, 5 of which were probably or definitely related to treatment.[61]

Indeed, research suggests that the risk of AE diminishes over multiple treatment sessions. In a multicenter study of 65 subjects who received regular BTX-A injections for hemifacial spasm over 10 years, Defazio and colleagues found that the incidence of AE decreased over time, falling from 37% during the first year of treatment to 12% in the tenth year.[62] In an analysis of 45 women who received continuous BTX-A injections for movement disorders for a mean duration of 15 years, recorded AE occurred in 35.6% and 22.2% of subjects at first and last visits, respectively.[63] Finally, Rzany and colleagues analyzed more than 4000 treatments in 945 people injected in the upper face and found only mild or moderate side effects, such as bruising and eyelid drooping, and side effects decreased with repeated injections.[64]

Complications

BTX works through temporary chemodenervation of the muscle, resulting in localized reduction of muscular activity. The authors believe that many complications can be avoided by using more concentrated doses, which allows for more accurate placement of BTX, less diffusion, and greater duration of effect.

Brow and eyelid ptosis lasting for up to 3 months are the most troublesome complications that can occur in the upper face, and both are caused by

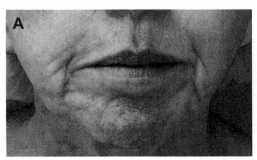
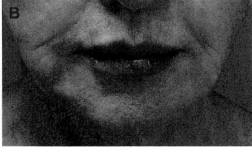

Fig. 5. Combination therapy in the lower face: before (A) and after treatment with BTX-A and hyaluronic acid (B).

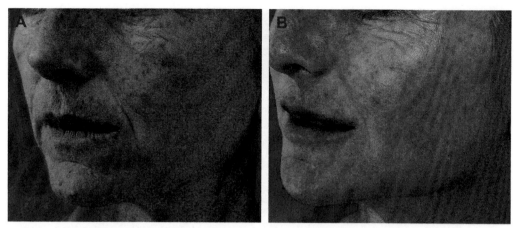

Fig. 6. Before (A) and after whole-face treatment with Intense Pulsed Light, BTX-A into the depressor anguli oris, mentalis, and orbicularis, plus concomitant treatment with soft-tissue augmentation of the melolabial, nasolabial, and malar regions (B).

diffusion of the toxin into adjacent musculature. The risk of brow ptosis, which is caused by product diffusion into the frontalis, can be avoided by preinjecting the brow depressors, avoiding preexisting brow ptosis, and injecting the glabella and forehead in separate treatment sessions.[56] Similarly, eyelid ptosis occurs when BTX-A injections into the glabella affect the upper eyelid levator muscle by way of diffusion. Higher concentrations, careful placement of the toxin (1 cm above the bony orbital rim, 1.5 cm lateral to the lateral canthus), and advising patients to refrain from manipulating the treated area for several hours after injection can help avoid eyelid ptosis. Other complications that have been reported include cocked eyebrow, diplopia, ectropion, asymmetrical smile, decreased strength of eye closure, and dry eye.[56]

In the lower face, complications are usually caused by overenthusiastic use of large doses, and can include mouth incompetence, asymmetry, drooling, difficulties in speech, and the inability to purse the lips.[56] Small doses of BTX-A injected superficially and symmetrically can decrease the potential for complications, as can placement; injections too close to the mouth or directly into the mental fold or orbicularis oris are more likely to result in undesirable effects (eg, flaccid cheek, incompetent mouth, or asymmetric smile). In the neck, large doses of BTX-A can lead to difficulty swallowing and general weakness.

Immunogenicity and Allergic Response

Antibody formation rarely occurs in current lots of BTX-A, which contain lower total protein loads than earlier formulations (prior to 1998), but has

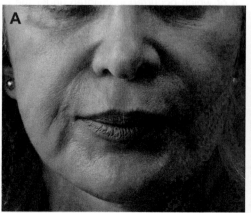
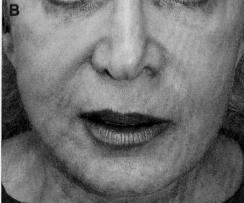

Fig. 7. Before (A) and after whole-face treatment with Intense Pulsed Light, BTX-A into the depressor anguli oris, mentalis, and orbicularis oris, and soft-tissue augmentation of the nasojugal folds, malar fat pads, nasolabial folds, melomental folds, and chin (B).

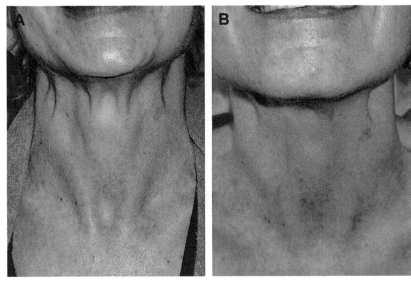

Fig. 8. Before (*A*) and after treatment of the platysma with BTX-A (*B*).

been reported, particularly when large doses are injected (eg, those associated with therapeutic applications).[63,65] Although the overall risk of antibody formation is low when using the lowest possible dose with the longest feasible intervals between injections,[66] a recent report describes an unusual case of a 20-year-old patient who developed antibody-induced therapy failure after the fourth injection series in the frontalis (60 U per session, 4 to 5 months between treatments).[67] Circulating antibodies against BTX-A were detected by indirect enzyme-linked immunosorbent assay and mouse protection assay.

Similarly, allergic reaction to BTX-A is rare but can be found in the literature. Reported reactions include serious or nonserious rashes[57,68] and granulomas.[69] Other allergic responses include a localized anaphylactic reaction in one leg,[68] a case of anaphylaxis after injection of BTX-A and lidocaine for the treatment of chronic neck and back pain,[70] and one patient who experienced severe respiratory failure after leg injections of 300 U BTX-A.[71]

Serious Adverse Events: Therapeutic Botulinum Toxin-A

A large examination of 1031 AE reports submitted to the FDA revealed 36 classified as serious for cosmetic BTX-A (headaches, facial paralysis, muscle weakness, dysphagia, flu like symptoms, and allergic reactions).[57] Of those 36, 13 had underlying disease that may have contributed to the reported AE, and serious AE were most common with significantly higher doses associated with therapeutic BTX-A. Indeed, the 407 AE

reported to the FDA for the therapeutic use of BTX-A (median dose, 100 U) included 28 deaths and other serious AE, such as arrhythmia and myocardial infarction. However, the report could not determine a causal relationship between the fatalities and BTX-A injections, especially since 26 patients who died had underlying cardiovascular diseases with an elevated risk of mortality. No deaths or cardiovascular complications were reported after treatment with significantly lower cosmetic doses.

In early 2008, the national consumer advocacy group, Public Citizen, petitioned the FDA to warn the public about serious side effects associated with BTX after analyzing FDA data that included 658 AE, of which 180 were aspiration, dysphagia, or pneumonia.[72] There were 16 deaths reported, 4 of which occurred in children under the age of 18. In response, the FDA announced a pending safety review focusing on high-dose therapeutic uses of BTX.[73] The review involves a small number of AE reports and large doses in patients with juvenile cerebral palsy and other lower-limb spasticities; none of the AE relate to a death as a result of cosmetic BTX-A.

Other reports have called the safety of BTX-A into question. Media announcements of death or paralysis after injection of cosmetic BTX-A were ultimately found to be the result of fake products that are unapproved, untested, and of questionable content.[74,75] In 2008, Antonucci and colleagues[76] injected BTX-A into the whisker muscles of rats and mice and found trace amounts of the toxin in the brainstem three days later. However, the BTX-A used in the study was an uncomplexed toxin (150,000 kDa molecule) produced in the laboratory for veterinarian research purposes and is not approved for human use by any governing body, and the doses used were up to 10 times higher than approved doses to treat glabellar rhytides in humans (translating into up to 150 times higher per kilogram/body weight).

SUMMARY

Botulinum toxins have been used therapeutically in humans for nearly 30 years and carry an impressive record of efficacy and safety when used appropriately. Originally used for the treatment of simple rhytides in the upper face, BTX-A is used to sculpt and mould the face into more pleasing contours, and is now considered an integral component of facial rejuvenation and an adjunct to other cosmetic surgical and nonsurgical procedures. Side effects are mostly mild and transient; more serious complications and AE are caused by poor injection technique or doses that are too large in already medically compromised patients. With the tiny amounts of BTX used for cosmetic applications, complications are usually local and related to injection technique. In addition, systemic complications virtually never occur because of the smaller doses necessary for cosmetic applications. Careful adherence to product, dosing, and placement can do much for the avoidance of more serious AE. Indeed, it is the authors' prediction that the uses of BTX and development of new products will only continue to grow in the next few years.

REFERENCES

1. Schantz EJ. Historical perspective. In: Jankovic J, Hallet M, editors. Therapy with botulinum toxin. New York: Marcel Dekker Inc.; 1994.
2. Schantz EJ, Johnson EA. Preparation and characterization of botulinum toxin type A for human treatment. In: Jankovic J, Hallet M, editors. Therapy with botulinum toxin. New York: Marcel Dekker Inc.; 1994.
3. Scott AB. Botulinum toxin injection into extraocular muscles as an alternative to strabismus surgery. Ophthalmology 1980;87:1044–9.
4. Carruthers JDA, Carruthers JA. Treatment of glabellar frown lines with C. Botulinum A exotoxin. J Dermatol Surg Oncol 1992;18:17–21.
5. Borodic GE, Cheney M, McKenna M. Contralateral injections of botulinum A toxin for the treatment of hemifacial spasm to achieve increased facial symmetry. Plast Reconstr Surg 1992;90:972–7.
6. Blitzer A, Brin MF, Keen MS, et al. Botulinum toxin for the treatment of hyperfunctional lines of the face. Arch Otolaryngol Head Neck Surg 1993;119: 1018–22.
7. Carruthers J, Carruthers A. The evolution of botulinum neurotoxin type A for cosmetic applications. J Cosmet Laser Ther 2007;9:186–92.
8. Carruthers A, Carruthers J. Botulinum toxin products overview. Skin Therapy Lett 2008;13:1–4.
9. Lowe PL, Patnaik R, Lowe NJ. A comparison of two botulinum type A toxin preparations for the treatment of glabellar lines: double-blind, randomized, pilot study. Dermatol Surg 2005;31:1651–4.
10. Trindade de Almeida AR, Marques E, de Almeida J, et al. Pilot study comparing the diffusion of two formulations of botulinum toxin type A in patients with forehead hyperhidrosis. Dermatol Surg 2007; 33(1 Spec No.):S37–43.
11. Cliff SH, Judodihardjo H, Eltringham E. Different formulations of botulinum toxin type A have different migration characteristics: a double-blind, randomized study. J Cosmet Dermatol 2008;7: 50–4.
12. Karsai S, Raulin C. Current evidence on the unit equivalence of different botulinum neurotoxin A formulations and recommendations for clinical practice in dermatology. Dermatol Surg 2009;35: 1–8.
13. Kranz G, Haubenberger D, Voller B, et al. Respective potencies of Botox(R) and Dysport(R) in a human skin model: a randomized, double-blind study. Mov Disord 2009;24:231–6.
14. Dressler D. [Pharmacological aspects of therapeutic botulinum toxin preparations]. Nervenarzt 2006;77: 912–21 [in German].
15. Roggenkamper P, Jost WH, Bihari K, et al. Efficacy and safety of a new botulinum toxin type A free of complexing proteins in the treatment of blepharospasm. J Neural Transm 2006;113:303–12.
16. Jost WH, Blumel J, Grafe S. Botulinum neurotoxin type A free of complexing proteins (XEOMIN) in focal dystonia. Drugs 2007;67:669–83.
17. Spencer JM, Gordon M, Goldberg DJ. Botulinum B treatment of the glabellar and frontalis regions: a dose response analysis. J Cosmet Laser Ther 2002;4:19–23.
18. Jacob CI. Botulinum neurotoxin type B–a rapid wrinkle reducer. Semin Cutan Med Surg 2003;22: 131–5.
19. Flynn TC, Clark RE. Botulinum toxin type B (MYOBLOC) versus botulinum type A (BOTOX) frontalis study: rate of onset and radius of diffusion. Dermatol Surg 2003;29:519–22.
20. Tang X, Wan X. Comparison of botox with a Chinese type A botulinum toxin. Chin Med J 2000;113:794–8.
21. Hunt T, Clarke K. Potency of the botulinum toxin product CNBTX-A significantly exceeds labeled

units in standard potency test. J Am Acad Dermatol 2008;58:517–8.

22. Stone AV, Ma J, Whitlock PW, et al. Effects of botox and neuronox on muscle force generation in mice. J Orthop Res 2007;25:1658–64.

23. Carruthers A, Carruthers J. Botulinum toxin type A: history and current cosmetic use in the upper face. Semin Cutan Med Surg 2001;20:71–84.

24. Carruthers J, Carruthers A. Botulinum toxin A in the mid and lower face and neck. Dermatol Clin 2004; 22:151–8.

25. Lowe NJ, Yamauchi P. Cosmetic uses of botulinum toxins for lower aspects of the face and neck. Clin Dermatol 2004;22:18–22.

26. Dayan SH, Maas CS. Botulinum toxins for facial wrinkles: beyond glabellar lines. Facial Plast Surg Clin North Am 2007;15:41–9.

27. Kaplan SE, Sherris DA, Gassner HG, et al. The use of botulinum toxin A in perioral rejuvenation. Facial Plast Surg Clin North Am 2007;15:415–21.

28. Fagien S, Carruthers JD. A comprehensive review of patient-reported satisfaction with botulinum toxin type a for aesthetic procedures. Plast Reconstr Surg 2008;122:1915–25.

29. Frankel AS, Kamer FM. Chemical browlift. Arch Otolaryngol Head Neck Surg 1998;124:321–3.

30. Huilgol S, Carruthers JA, Carruthers JDA. Raising eyebrows with botulinum toxin. Dermatol Surg 1999;25:373–6.

31. Carruthers A, Carruthers J. Eyebrow height after botulinum toxin type A to the glabella. Dermatol Surg 2007;33:26–32.

32. Flynn TC, Carruthers JA, Carruthers JA. Botulinum-A toxin treatment of the lower eyelid improves infraorbital rhytides and widens the eye. Dermatol Surg 2001;27:703–8.

33. Flynn TC, Carruthers JA, Carruthers JA, et al. Botulinum A toxin (BOTOX) in the lower eyelid: dose-finding study. Dermatol Surg 2003;29:943–50.

34. To EW, Ahuja AT, Ho WS, et al. A prospective study of the effect of botulinum toxin A on masseteric muscle hypertrophy with ultrasonographic and electromyographic measurement. Br J Plast Surg 2001; 54:197–200.

35. von Lindern JJ, Niederhagen B, Appel T, et al. Type A botulinum toxin for the treatment of hypertrophy of the masseter and temporal muscle: an alternative treatment. Plast Reconstr Surg 2001; 107:327–32.

36. Park MY, Ahn KY, Jung DS. Application of botulinum toxin A for treatment of facial contouring in the lower face. Dermatol Surg 2003;29:477–83.

37. Kim NH, Chung JH, Park RH, et al. The use of botulinum toxin type A in aesthetic mandibular contouring. Plast Reconstr Surg 2005;115:919–30.

38. Liew S, Dart A. Nonsurgical reshaping of the lower face. Aesthet Surg J 2008;28:251–7.

39. Tartaro G, Rauso R, Santagata M, et al. Lower facial contouring with botulinum toxin type A. J Craniofac Surg 2008;19:1613–7.

40. Chikhani L, Dichamp J. [Bruxism, temporo-mandibular dysfunction and botulinum toxin]. Ann Readapt Med Phys 2003;46:333–7 [in French].

41. Fagien S. Botox for the treatment of dynamic and hyperkinetic facial lines and furrows: adjunctive use in facial aesthetic surgery. Plast Reconstr Surg 1999;103:701–13.

42. Fagien S, Brandt FS. Primary and adjunctive use of botulinum toxin type A (botox) in facial aesthetic surgery: beyond the glabella. Clin Plast Surg 2001; 28:127–48.

43. Carruthers J, Carruthers A. A prospective, randomized, parallel group study analyzing the effect of BTX-A(botox) and nonanimal sourced hyaluronic acid (NASHA, restylane) in combination compared with NASHA (restylane) alone in severe glabellar rhytides in adult female subjects: treatment of severe glabellar rhytides with a hyaluronic acid derivative compared with the derivative and BTX-A. Dermatol Surg 2003;29:802–9.

44. Coleman KR, Carruthers J. Combination therapy with BOTOX and fillers: the new rejuvenation paradigm. Dermatol Ther 2006;19:177–88.

45. Carruthers J, Carruthers A, Maberley D. Deep resting glabellar rhytides respond to BTX-A and Hylan B. Dermatol Surg 2003;29:539–44.

46. Patel MP, Talmor M, Nolan WB. Botox and collagen for glabellar furrows: advantages of combination therapy. Ann Plast Surg 2004;52:442–7.

47. Carruthers J, Carruthers A. The adjunctive usage of botulinum. Dermatol Surg 1998;24:1244–7.

48. West TB, Alster TS. Effect of botulinum toxin type A on movement-associated rhytides following CO_2 laser resurfacing. Dermatol Surg 1999;25:259–61.

49. Zimbler MS, Holds JB, Kokoska MS, et al. Effect of botulinum toxin pretreatment on laser resurfacing results: a prospective, randomized, blinded trial. Arch Facial Plast Surg 2001;3:165–9.

50. Carruthers J, Carruthers A. The effect of full-face broadband light treatments alone and in combination with bilateral crow's feet botulinum toxin type A chemodenervation. Dermatol Surg 2004;30: 355–66.

51. Khoury JG, Saluja R, Goldman MP. The effect of botulinum toxin type A on full-face intense pulsed light treatment: a randomized, double-blind, split-face study. Dermatol Surg 2008;34:1062–9.

52. Sherris DA, Gassner HG. Botulinum toxin to minimize facial scarring. Facial Plast Surg 2002;18: 35–9.

53. Gassner HG, Brissett AE, Otley CC, et al. Botulinum toxin to improve facial wound healing: a prospective, blinded, placebo-controlled study. Mayo Clin Proc 2006;81:1023–8.

54. Wilson AM. Use of botulinum toxin type A to prevent widening of facial scars. Plast Reconstr Surg 2006; 117:1758–66.

55. Alam M, Dover JS, Klein AW, et al. Botulinum A exotoxin for hyperfunctional facial lines: where not to inject. Arch Dermatol 2002;138:1180.

56. Klein AW. Complications, adverse reactions, and insights with the use of botulinum toxin. Dermatol Surg 2003;29:549–56.

57. Coté TR, Mohan AK, Polder JA, et al. Botulinum toxin type A injections: adverse events reported to the US Food and Drug Administration in therapeutic and cosmetic cases. J Am Acad Dermatol 2005;53:407–15.

58. Zagui RM, Matayoshi S, Moura FC. [Adverse effects associated with facial application of botulinum toxin: a systematic review with meta-analysis]. Arq Bras Oftalmol 2008;71:894–901 [in Portuguese].

59. Hsiung GY, Das SK, Ranawaya R, et al. Long-term efficacy of botulinum toxin A in treatment of various movement disorders over a 10-year period. Mov Disord 2002;17:1288–93.

60. Naumann M, Jankovic J. Safety of botulinum toxin type A: a systematic review and meta-analysis. Curr Med Res Opin 2004;20:981–90.

61. Carruthers J, Carruthers A. Complications of botulinum toxin A. Facial Plast Surg Clin North Am 2007;15:51–4.

62. Defazio G, Abbruzzese G, Girlanda P, et al. Botulinum toxin A treatment for primary hemifacial spasm: a 10-year multicenter study. Arch Neurol 2002;59:418–20.

63. Mejia NI, Vuong KD, Jankovic J. Long-term botulinum toxin efficacy, safety, and immunogenicity. Mov Disord 2005;20:592–7.

64. Rzany B, Dill-Müller D, Grablowitz D, et al. Repeated botulinum toxin A injections for the treatment of lines in the upper face: a retrospective study of 4,103 treatments in 945 patients. Dermatol Surg 2007; 33(1 Spec No.):S18–25.

65. Jankovic J, Vuong KD, Ahsan J. Comparison of efficacy and immunogenicity of original versus current botulinum toxin in cervical dystonia. Neurology 2003;60:1186–8.

66. Allergan, Inc. Botox cosmetic (botulinum toxin type A) purified neurotoxin complex (prescribing information). Irvine (CA): Allergan, Inc; 2005.

67. Lee SK. Antibody-induced failure of botulinum toxin type A therapy in a patient with masseteric hypertrophy. Dermatol Surg 2007;33(1 Spec No.): S105–10.

68. LeWitt PA, Trosch RM. Idiosyncratic adverse reactions to intramuscular botulinum toxin type A injection. Mov Disord 1997 Nov;12:1064–7.

69. Ahbib S, Lachapelle JM, Marot L. [Sarcoidal granulomas following injections of botulic toxin A (Botox) for corrections of wrinkles]. Ann Dermatol Venereol 2006;133:43–5 [in French].

70. Li M, Goldberger BA, Hopkins C. Fatal case of BOTOX-related anaphylaxis? J Forensic Sci 2005;50: 169–72.

71. Nong LB, He WQ, Xu YH, et al. [Severe respiratory failure after injection of botulinum toxin: case report and review of the literature]. Zhonghua Jie He He Hu Xi Za Zhi 2008;31:369–71 [in Chinese].

72. Public Citizen. Stricter warnings needed for botox, myobloc injections. Available at: http://www.citizen.org/pressroom/release.cfm?ID=2593. Accessed February 6, 2009.

73. U.S. Food and Drug Administration. Early communication about an ongoing safety review botox and botox cosmetic (botulinum toxin type A) and myobloc (botulinum toxin type B). Plast Surg Nurs 2008;28: 150–1.

74. USA TODAY 219 doctors purchase Botox knockoff. Available at: http://www.usatoday.com/news/health/2005-02-21-fake-botox-usat_x.htm. Accessed February 6, 2009.

75. The Business Edition. Woman dies from fake Botox injections. Available at: http://www.thebusinessedition.com/woman-dies-from-fake-botox-injections-213/#more-213. Accessed February 6, 2009.

76. Antonucci F, Rossi C, Gianfranceschi L, et al. Long-distance retrograde effects of botulinum neurotoxin A. J Neurosci 2008;28:3689–96.

Dermal Fillers and Combinations of Fillers for Facial Rejuvenation

Kenneth Beer, MD, PA

KEYWORDS

- Facial rejuvenation • Poly L lactic acid
- Calcium hydroxylapatite • Porcine collagen
- Silicone • Hyaluronic acid

Until recently, the use of dermal fillers was limited in the United States by the small number of products approved by the Food and Drug Administration (FDA). This limitation mandated that combinations of fillers frequently married an older technology, such as a human or bovine-derived collagen, with a newer product, such as a tightly cross-linked hyaluronic acid (HA). Although this methodology had its proponents who espoused the benefits of the lidocaine found in the collagens or the structure provided by collagen fibrils, the sheer lack of data combined with the want of results spelled the demise of these combinations. More recently, the products approved for use in the United States have opened up the range of possibilities for combinations of products that are synergistic in their effects. Combinations of products may be discussed in temporal or anatomic relationships. Temporal combinations refer to the use of different fillers at different times, whereas anatomic combinations refer to the use of different fillers in different parts of the face. Before discussing how the various fillers may be used in combination, it is worthwhile to consider their use in isolation. Soft-tissue augmentation products under consideration in the present article include the hyaluronic acids, poly L lactic acid (PLLA), calcium hydroxylapatite (CAHA), porcine collagen, and silicone.

HA are the most widely used soft-tissue augmentation products.[1] These molecules are polymers of d-glucuronic and n-acetyl-d-glycosamine, which are then cross-linked for stability following injection. The various products differ in their concentrations of cross-linked HA, degree of cross linkage, flow characteristics, tissue-lifting ability, and method of particle manufacture. In addition, some products contain lidocaine. The main HA products approved for use in the United States are those of the Restylane, Juvederm, and Prevelle families. Each has unique characteristics that affect their utility for specific indications and each has brand-extension products that will enhance the opportunities for combination treatments.

Collagens presently approved for use in the United States are porcine in nature. Autologous collagen (Isolagen) has not been demonstrated to be safe and effective, whereas bovine and human-derived collagens are not effective enough to warrant continued marketing and distribution. The porcine collagen used in the United States is Evolence, which has a novel ribose cross-linking technology.[2] This cross-linking is free from the types of chemical structures that appear foreign to the immune system, and thus, it has a longer duration of correction. Evolence is approved for 6 months duration and animal models suggest that this duration could be for as long as 9 to12 months.[3]

Evolence is unique in several aspects. Unlike the HA, it is opaque, and thus, is not suitable for placement in the superficial dermis. Because it contains collagen fibers, it is capable of providing some structural support but is less structural than Perlane or Radiesse. Although Evolence is not suited

Department of Dermatology, University of Miami, The Cosmetic Bootcamp, 1500 North Dixie Highway, Suite 303, West Palm Beach, FL 33401, USA
E-mail address: kenbeer@aol.com

Dermatol Clin 27 (2009) 427–432
doi:10.1016/j.det.2009.08.011
0733-8635/09/$ – see front matter © 2009 Elsevier Inc. All rights reserved.

for injections into the lip, a future version (Evolence Breeze) has smaller collagen chains and is approved for use in the lips outside of the United States.

The most logical uses for Evolence in isolation are to correct moderate depth nasolabial creases and marionette lines. As previously mentioned, its opaque nature make it less than ideal for superficial placement, but it is reasonable to combine it with HA, which can be placed superficially to it. Thus, Evolence may be used to replace volume in the marionette and nasolabial creases and a hyaluronic acid can be used to etch out the lines above the crease.

PLLA is a device capable of stimulating collagen production following its injection. It is suited for volume restoration. Its method of action relies upon stimulation of fibroblasts and other cells to lay down a matrix of collagen and elastic fibers.[4] Unlike many other devices, PLLA relies upon the physician to determine its ultimate formulation. Because it is a lyophilized powder, there remain many variables in its final concentration. According to the package insert, the recommended amount of water for each bottle is 3 to 5 mL.[5] In addition, the product requires at least 4 hours of time to imbibe water and become saturated. However, many experienced injectors of PLLA believe that leaving it in water for at least 24 hours is ideal. There is also considerable debate about the optimal reconstitution formulation for PLLA. Some advocate the use of 7 mL of water as diluent and others recommend that additional volume in the form of lidocaine be added into the mix. At the present time, there are few well-controlled clinical trials to determine what the optimal dilution or reconstitution formulae are.

Two areas uniquely suited for treatment with PLLA are the temporal and malar regions. As the malar fat pad becomes atrophic and descends, the middle third of the face becomes concave. Several malar grading scales are available to help assess the degree of malar descent and atrophy but the senior author believes that the SOBER scale is the most useful.[6] Injections into these areas should use dilutions of between 7 to 9 mL of fluid per bottle and it is recommended that dilution lasts for at least 24 hours. The addition of 2 mL of lidocaine with 1:100,000 epinephrine to 5 mL of water is helpful in decreasing patients' discomfort.

Injections of PLLA should be made at intervals of not less than 4 weeks, which enables the injector to minimize the risk of overcorrection and of subcutaneous papule formation. A 0.5 inch, 26-gauge needle may be inserted into the deep dermis or into the dermal/subcutaneous junction. It is better to inject PLLA into a deeper plane than a superficial one as the latter will result in the formation of papules. Multiple modalities of injection techniques are useful when injecting this product. Serial puncture, fanning, and linear threading may all be used to lay down a matrix of product in a deep plane. Because it is a suspended particle, rather than a homogenous solution, it can precipitate in the syringes so it is essential to inject in a rapid manner.

Malar injections should begin with one bottle of PLLA and typically require three or four bottles of product to correct moderate malar atrophy. Once the cheeks have been restored, it is reasonable to correct nasolabial creases, marionette lines, glabella furrows, atrophic lips, and perioral rhytids. None of these is best treated with PLLA. Thus, for many patients, the addition of another product will optimize the outcome. Depending on the anatomy and goals of patients, a hyaluron, collagen, or CAHA can be used to treat the discrete lines and creases. Patients that have fine lines or wrinkles in addition to their volume loss may have their nasolabial creases, marionette lines, or glabella treated with collagen or HA. Deeper folds may be treated with thick HA, such as Perlane, or with CAHA.

The use of CAHA for soft-tissue augmentation has been well documented, especially for use in the midface region.[7] Radiesse has been safely and effectively used to fill deep creases and to restore lost volume. Its use with other products, such as HA or collagen of different sized particles, is likely to increase in frequency as their utility become studied. Radiesse is of particular use for areas, such as the jaw, where bone resorption has played a dominant role in facial recession. CAHA has been injected in a variety of locations, and to date, there are two areas of the face that should be avoided. One area that should not be injected with CAHA is the vermillion of the lip because of the increased rate of nodule formation in this location. Another area that may be best served by other fillers is the tear trough, where injections may lead to visible nodules that are apparent through the thin skin of this location.

HA products may be combined with each other and with other classes of fillers. There are many different rationales for the combinations, which are primarily based upon their structural and flow characteristics. Juvederm has several attributes that render it very smooth and easily injected. Thus, it is a good candidate for the treatment of the tear troughs and of lip atrophy. Patients that have superficial perioral rhytids may also benefit from Juvederm injections.

However, it does not have the lifting or structural qualities of other fillers and may not be suitable for malar injections.

COMBINATIONS FOR FACIAL REJUVENATION

The most interesting development in the arena of facial rejuvenation is not the advent of any single product or technology but rather the possibilities of combining the various treatments and products in ways heretofore not possible. For instance, addressing midface descent with injections into the malar area can help lift the face, but if there are static perioral lines and the malar fat pad has evaporated, there will not be a symmetry or balance to the face. The ability to use soft products in the lips and perioral areas, firm products for sculpting, volumizers for volume restoration, botulinum toxins in dynamic areas, and lasers and light sources on the surface and mid dermal structures is by far the most significant development in recent history. As we learn more about individual products, we will gain more insights into their use with each other. For now, however, it is useful to have some rational framework to consider which combinations make sense for restoring facial anatomy to a more youthful appearance. In broad terms, we may divide products into those that add volume, those that fill lines, those that provide lift, and those that are able to buttress. There is a broad overlap with product indications and none is limited to one of these categories by either the FDA or their intrinsic properties. However, it is useful to begin to think about fillers in this manner to help devise methodologies that provide optimal outcomes for patients.

VOLUMIZERS WITH FILLERS

Many, if not most, patients that have lost enough volume to benefit from PLLA will also need treatment of lines that have developed. PLLA has an excellent safety and efficacy profile when used for volume restoration. The areas that are still in a state of flux are the proper amount, type of diluent, and timing of reconstitution used. Originally, reconstitution with water was recommended for at least 4 hours before use and with a 3 mL quantity. This has since changed and many injectors are using more water, more time, and adding in lidocaine with 1:100,000 epinephrine. There has not been a definitive clinical trial to support any dilution or methodology, and for now it is reasonable to use 4 mL of water for more than 24 hours to reconstitute the product. Immediately before use, the senior author adds an additional 3 to 4 mL of 1% lidocaine with 1:100,000 epinephrine (if patients have epinephrine sensitivity or are elderly, this may be deleted).

Optimal combinations using volumizers with fillers are ones that address the issues in a coherent manner. Among the most common are PLLA in the cheeks, lower jaw, and temples, with fillers in the cheeks, marionette, and perioral areas. This strategy offers the core physician the opportunity to demonstrate mastery of facial rejuvenation and offers the patients the benefit of the use of products that excel at specific functions for defined locations.

Many patients lose volume of the malar and temporal areas beginning at approximately 50 years of age. This anatomic shift has been documented by Rohrich and Pessal.[8] Restoration of the temporal and malar areas may be achieved with PLLA. To begin this process, patients need to have a thorough understanding that treatments with PLLA are a process rather than a discrete procedure and that several injection sessions are planned. As with any procedure, the risks, benefits, and alternatives of this treatment should be discussed. For PLLA, one unique potential adverse event is the formation of subcutaneous papules, with an estimated incidence of approximately 2%.[9] Injections of PLLA should be made with a 25- or 26-gauge needle that is between 0.5 to 1 in. When administering PLLA to the malar area, the goal should be to lay down a three-dimensional matrix of product that will stimulate collagen production in a uniform manner. However, since one is injecting a particulate product suspended in a liquid medium (rather than a gel) the reality is that despite one's best attempts to place the product homogenously, its distribution is subject to gravitational, muscular, and thermal forces before it begins its collagen stimulation.

Adding volume to the malar area should begin with one bottle of material injected at the dermal/subcutaneous plane. When injecting, particularly in people with thin skin, it is preferable to err on the side of deep placement rather than superficial. For patients with a concavity, the goal should be restoration of a normal contour with PLLA. A cross hatching technique is recommended for treating this location as it enables the product to disperse evenly throughout the tissue planes. It is also advisable to inject the product with some degree of cross hatching to ensure that there is adequate dispersion of the product along the desired plane. Treatments should be spaced at 1-month intervals with approximately three treatments planned before a rest interval of a few weeks is taken to measure the response.

Concomitant with the depletion of malar soft tissue, there is frequent loss of temporal soft tissue. Treatment of this area is also ideally suited to injections with PLLA. These treatments should use one bottle per session for most patients and may be performed at the same time as the malar treatments. A 1-inch needle is preferred for this treatment as injections should be performed at the plane just superior to the periosteum (deep to the muscular layer). A linear threading and fanning technique may be used to deposit PLLA in this plane.

PLLA is also being increasingly used to treat the prejowl sulcus. This area is a frequent source of cosmetic concern as the loss of underlying bone and soft tissue depletes the support for the overlying skin and the corners of the mouth. Injections of this area may be approached from the inferior aspect of the ramus. When injecting this location, one must be cautious to avoid the underlying vasculature. A fanning technique may be used to deposit 0.5 cc of PLLA on each side. Over time, as volume is restored, it is possible to attain reshaping of this area to a more youthful appearance. One additional benefit is that by restoring volume here, it is easier to address some of the other concerns that affect the mouth and perioral areas.

Addressing additional stigmata of facial aging may be performed at the same time as volume correction with PLLA. PLLA may help not only to restore youthful contours to the temple, cheeks, and prejowl areas but also the appearance of the skin. Some fine lines that traverse the cheeks will fade with PLLA treatments. However, many lines that are in other areas will remain unaffected and require injections with other products or treatments with lasers.

Treatment of moderate to severe nasolabial creases can be effected with several products approved for the treatment of this area. Selection of the product used for this purpose depends on patients' skin type, skin thickness, tolerance for risk, goals, and budget. Evolence, Restylane, Perlane, Juvederm, Juvederm XC, and Radiesse are all products that will do well in this area. When injecting patients who have thin skin and moderate rhytids, it is wise to inject a clear hyaluron gel for the first injections. This is even truer when the product will be placed closer to the epidermis to etch out lines. Thicker, opaque products, such as Evolence and Radiesse, offer the potential to have longer-term corrections with a single injection session, but have adverse events that are potentially more long lived and more difficult to manage than the hyalurons. Thus, they are more appropriate for advanced injectors or for patients that have been treated previously. When combined with PLLA injections of the cheeks, average patients will require approximately 2 mL of filler in the nasolabial creases.

Perioral rhytids are a frequent companion of malar volume loss. Treatment of these lines with PLLA is inappropriate as it will lead to a high rate of subcutaneous papules. However, treating these lines with botulinum toxins, lasers, and fillers may produce dramatic results. For the majority of patients who have moderate to severe perioral rhytids, injections with hyaluronic acid will produce significant improvements. Products well suited for this indication include Prevelle, which is also short lived and useful as a test product for this indication, Juvederm, and Restylane. The addition of 1 to 2 units of Botox or 2.5 to 5 units of Reloxin for hypertrophic orbicularis muscles may help to improve these lines.[10] For some patients, even after fillers are used, it is useful to have the surface of the skin polished with either a fractional ablative or fractional nonablative laser. Since the perioral area is a center of attention, it is reasonable to use combinations of treatments to address it and to treat this area in conjunction with treatments of other areas.

Fillers are also helpful in treating superficial marionette lines. Thus, it is possible to restore volume in the prejowl sulcus while having residual lines in the superficial and mid dermis. Restoring this layer of correction with a volume filler is a rational complement to PLLA injections. Several products may be used to treat marionette lines with common ones including Juvederm, Restylane, Perlane, Evolence, and Radiesse. When injecting this area, one needs to be aware of the potential for product migration into the vermillion of the lip.[11]

FILLERS WITH FILLERS

The advent of so many fillers to the United States markets has brought possibilities for combinations that can achieve results that were not attainable with the limited selection available a few years ago. Intuitively, thick fillers that are structural may be used for deeper creases, whereas thinner products may be used to treat superficial lines closer to the epidermis. Fillers with anesthetic may be used to make areas more comfortable before injection of products without anesthetic.

The most obvious method of combining different fillers is either geographically or spatially, that is, using different products in different locations or different products at different times. Thus, patients that have had a positive outcome from a short-lived HA may get a longer-term product injected at a subsequent visit. The initial

HA will most likely still be extant and the combination will likely produce some synergy. Geographic combinations are another common injection strategy. Largely based on anecdotal evidence and personal experience, some fillers in the same category have become preferred for certain locations. Patients presenting for treatment of several facial issues may get Juvederm Ultra in the tear trough and UltraPlus in the lips, while getting Restylane in the nasolabial crease, and Perlane in the marionette lines.

In addition to temporal and geographic separation, products may be layered on each other or mixed together. Thus, structural fillers that are useful for deep-tissue filling or support include CAHA, Perlane, and to some extent, Evolence. Each of these may be used and has the ability to provide significant lifting. However, properties of each limit their utility for filling lines.

CAHA provides a matrix that provides initial correction with subsequent collagen and elastic tissue ingrowth that helps to support the overlying structures. However, it is an opaque, white product that can be visualized when placed too close to the epidermis. In addition, when injected in the superficial dermis, it may produce nodules. Although it is suitable for deep-tissue placement, it is not appropriate for superficial line filling. However, combinations of this product with other fillers can address both facets of the aging face. Products that may be layered above CAHA include Restylane, Juvederm, and Prevelle. Each of these may be injected superficially with a 30-gauge needle to lift the wrinkle away from the underlying CAHA and to fill the superficial lines. Which of these is selected depends on a variety of factors including the thickness of the skin and the physician's experiences. Each may be injected with a linear threading, serial puncture, or a combination of techniques.

Combinations of hyaluronic acids can also be used to optimize patients' results. For instance, different hyalurons may be used to treat different parts of the anatomy or they may be layered upon each other. Injections into the tear troughs and lips require different properties than structural lifting of the zygoma. For the tear trough and lips, patients who have thin skin may benefit from injections with Juvederm. However, these patients may require more Perlane for their marionette lines or Restylane for their nasolabial creases. Additional combinations include the intermarriage of Perlane injections into the deep layer for volume, or contour correction with Juvederm, or Restylane injected superficially to smooth the superficial layers. Temporal combinations may also benefit certain patients. For instance, some patients that

are injected with one filler may return for an enhancement procedure. These enhancements are typically performed with the same product that was originally injected. However, there are instances where a thicker, more structural hyaluron must be injected deep to the prior injection to change the contour, and other circumstances where a softer product may be layered superficially to the structural product to etch out a line that is the focus of the patients' attention. Although the literature demonstrates that enhancement injections with the same product results in a more durable correction (through mechanisms not yet defined), there is no reason to believe that this same phenomenon will not occur when different hyalurons are injected together.[12]

The areas that are commonly treated with these combinations are the nasolabial creases and the marionette lines. On average, a woman with moderate tissue loss of the nasolabial creases will require between 1 to 1.3 mL of Radiesse per nasolabial crease with about 0.5 mL of hyaluronic acid layered superficial to it. Marionette lines may be treated with less volume and many women can be effectively treated with 0.65 mL of Radiesse and about 0.5 mL of hyaluronic acid superficial to this. As with injections of single products, it is essential to inject the angles of the mouth with some hyaluronic acid to restore a horizontal projection to this area.

Evolence is an opaque, cross-linked porcine collagen that can also provide long lasting (up to 9–12 months) support for the marionette lines and nasolabial creases. Many nasolabial creases are adequately treated with 1 mL of Evolence on each side. Treatment of the marionette lines is also easily accomplished with Evolence. Average volumes for this treatment should begin with 0.5 mL on each side. However, as with Radiesse, one cannot place Evolence too close to the epidermis for risk of creating visible papules. Thus, it is helpful to layer a hyaluronic acid superficial to the Evolence when treating lines that have a superficial component in addition to the deeper loss of volume.

Silicone is a permanent soft-tissue augmentation product that is used in an off-label manner. It has been combined with various additives over the years, frequently with disastrous results.[13] Silicone has been inadvertently combined with numerous products as patients who had been treated with this agent in the past present for injections of additional products. Among the frequent combinations that occur are silicone with collagen and silicone with hyaluronic acid. Because silicone can cause granulomas, even after being dormant for many years, there is some potential for problems in areas that contain silicone. In addition, silicone may be encapsulated and present a flow barrier to soft-tissue augmentation products, such as hyaluronic acid. Thus, it is recommended that combinations of other soft-tissue augmentation products with silicone proceed gradually and that the risks and benefits be presented to patients before treatment. In some instances, fillers may be combined with silicone to mask a contour deformity created by this product.

SUMMARY

Soft-tissue augmentation has evolved enormously in the past few years and we are just learning optimal methods of using and combining products already on the market. Clearly, some of the products introduced have not been commercially accepted for reasons of safety, efficacy, or market demand and it is likely that many more products of dubious distinction will also be introduced. However, the vast majority of products used for soft-tissue augmentation will find niches in which they excel.

Whether we are using different types of HA, HA with collagen, PLLA with HA, or any of the other myriad of combinations available, we now have the ability to address the root causes of facial aging in a manner not even conceivable a few years ago. Truly, this is an interesting and exciting time to be in this specialty.

REFERENCES

1. ASAPS 2007 Data. Available at: www.surgery.com. Accessed June 12, 2009.
2. Narins R, Brandt FS, Lorenc ZP, et al. A randomized multicenter study of the safety and efficacy of dermicol P35 and non animal stabilized hyaluronic acid gel for the correction of nasolabial folds. Dermatol Surg 2007;33:S213–21.
3. Pitaru S, Noff M, Blok L, et al. Long term efficacy of a novel cross linked collagen dermal filler: a histologic and histomorphometric study in an animal model. Dermatol Surg 2007;33(9):1045–54.
4. Vleggar D, Bauer U. Facial enhancement and the European experience with Sculptra. J Drugs Dermatol 2004;3:542–7.
5. Sculptra Package Insert. Sanofi Aventis. Bridgewater, NJ.
6. Solish N, Beer K, Remington K. A Grading system for the malar crease region and its implications for treatment of this region with soft tissue augmentation products. Journal of Drugs in Dermatology 2008; 8(4):S4–7.
7. Graivier MH, Bass LS, Busso M, et al. Calcium hydroxylapatite (Radiesse) for correction of the mid and lower face: consensus recommendations. Plast Reconstr Surg 2007;120(6 Suppl):55S–66S.
8. Rohrich R, Pessa J. The fat components of the face: anatomy and clinical implications for cosmetic surgery. Plast Reconstr Surg 2007;119(12):2219.
9. Burgess CM, Quiroga RM. Assessment of the safety and efficacy of poly L lactic acid for the treatment of HIV associated facial lipoatrophy. J Am Acad Dermatol 2005;52:233–9.
10. Semchyshyn N, Sengelman RD. Botulinum a treatment of perioral rhytids. Dermatol Surg 2003;29(5): 490–5.
11. Beer K. Radiesse nodule of the lips from a distant injection site: report of a case and consideration of etiology and management. J Drugs Dermatol 2007; 6:829–30.
12. Wang F, Garza LA, Kang S, et al. In Vivo Stimulation of de novo collagen production caused by cross linked hyaluronic acid dermal filler injections in photodamaged human skin. Arch Dermatol 2007; 143(2):155–63.
13. Duffy D. Silicone conundrum: a battle of anecdotes. Dermatol Surg 2002;28(7):590–4.

Semipermanent and Permanent Injectable Fillers

Derek H. Jones, MD

KEYWORDS

- Semipermanent and permanent fillers
- Hyaluronic acid • Calcium hyaluronic polylactic acid
- Polymethyl methacrylate

Soft-tissue augmentation dates back more than 100 years ago, when autologous fat grafts were used to restore facial volume defects.[1] Paraffin was used for some time but fell out of favor because of a high incidence of foreign-body reactions. In the early 1950s, liquid silicone was first injected for soft-tissue augmentation. It was used widely until 1982, when the US Food and Drug Administration (FDA) temporarily banned its use over concerns of possible toxicity. Following the ban on liquid silicone, injectable bovine collagen became available in the United States in the 1980s and quickly became the gold standard of treatment to which many new dermal fillers are still compared. Although some may question the duration of effect of collagen, human collagen remains an agent of comparison in many pivotal trials.

Today, an impressive array of injectable dermal fillers for facial soft-tissue augmentation is available in the United States. These agents, most of which were introduced in the last half decade, represent a variety of semipermanent and permanent fillers across several categories. Physicians can choose between semipermanent fillers, such as hyaluronic acid derivatives (HA), calcium hydroxylapatite (CaHA), and poly-L-lactic acid (PLA), and longer-lasting, so-called "permanent fillers," such as polymethyl methacrylate microspheres (PMMA), highly purified forms of liquid silicone, and hydrogel polymers.

While these fillers are generally safe, effectiveness is related to areas of injection and physician expertise. Each has its own specific properties and longevity that makes it more suitable for certain uses than for others. Semipermanent fillers must be repeated at regular intervals, although with certain products the filler is replaced by the patients' own collagen over the course of several treatments. Permanent fillers require minimal touch-ups and have long-lasting effects of 5 years and longer.

SEMIPERMANENT FILLERS
Calcium Hydroxylapatite

CaHA is a normal component of human bone and teeth and has been used as implant or coating material in dentistry and other therapeutic areas for more than 20 years. The filler is composed of CaHA microspheres (25–45 microns) suspended in an aqueous carboxymethylcellulose gel carrier. Radiesse (Bio-Form Medical, San Mateo, California) is the dermal filler containing CaHA. Skin testing is not required.

Mechanism of action

The mechanical filling and volume enhancement occurs following injection, when the gel carrier and CaHA microspheres displace surrounding soft tissue. As the gel is phagocytized, the process of neocollagenesis begins in and around the microspheres, stimulating the gradual growth of the patients' own collagen (Fig. 1).[2] The spherical CaHA particles are gradually broken down and degraded by way of normal metabolic processes and eliminated as calcium and phosphate ions through the urinary system. The proliferation of collagen along with the slow breakdown of the CaHA is understood to account for the prolonged effects.[3]

Indications

CaHA is indicated for subdermal implantation for the correction of moderate to severe facial wrinkles

Skin Care and Laser Physicians of Beverly Hills, 9201 W. Sunset Boulevard, Suite 602, Los Angeles, CA 90069, USA
E-mail address: derekjonesmd@gmail.com

Dermatol Clin 27 (2009) 433–444
doi:10.1016/j.det.2009.08.003
0733-8635/09/$ – see front matter © 2009 Elsevier Inc. All rights reserved.

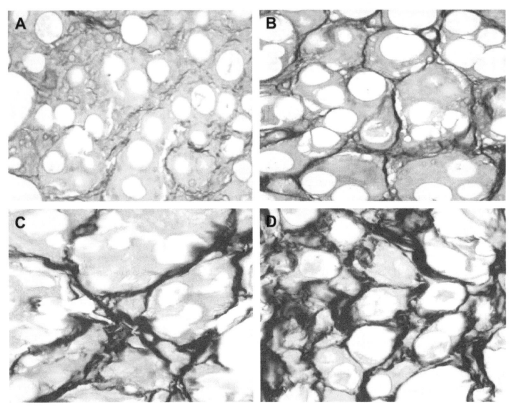

Fig. 1. (A–D) Histology studies demonstrate increased collagen deposition around CaHA microspheres over 4 to 78 weeks. Collagen fibers are represented by the darker areas. (*From* Coleman KM, Voights R, DeVore DP, et al. Neo-collagenesis after injection of calcium hydroxylapatite composition in a canine model. Dermatol Surg 2008;34:S53–5; with permission.)

and folds, including nasolabial folds (**Fig. 2**), and for the correction of HIV-associated facial lipoatrophy (**Fig. 3**). It is also indicated for vocal cord insufficiency, oral/maxillofacial defects, and radiographic tissue marking. Off-label facial uses also include correction of marionette lines and oral commissures, prejowl sulcus, cheek-volume loss, and dorsal nasal deformities. In its present formulation, CaHA is not appropriate for use in the lips.

Efficacy and safety

CaHA was compared with a human-collagen product in a United States pivotal trial of 117 subjects with moderate to severe nasolabial folds. These subjects were randomized to receive CaHA on one side of the face and an existing human collagen (HC) product (Cosmoplast, Inamed, Santa Barbara, California) on the other. CaHA provided significantly longer correction than HC,

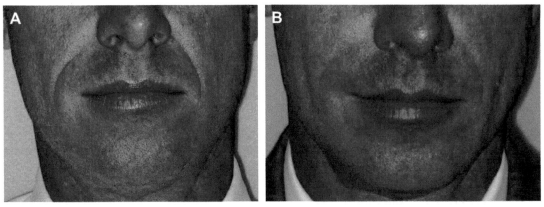

Fig. 2. (A, B) Pretreatment and posttreatment photographs of injection with Radiesse for nasolabial folds. Total volume injected into nasolabial folds was 1.3 mL. (*Courtesy of* D. Jones, MD, Los Angeles, CA.)

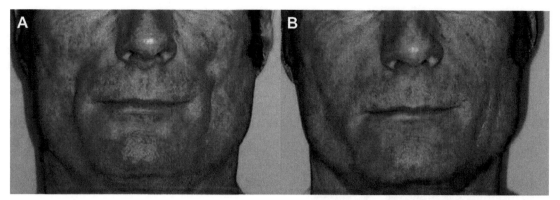

Fig. 3. (A, B) Pretreatment and posttreatment photographs of injection with Radiesse for HIV-associated facial lipoatrophy. (*Courtesy of* D. Jones, MD, Los Angeles.)

and the favorable adverse event profile was similar to HC.[4]

In this split-face study, the mean change in pretreatment score using the Lemperle Rating Scale over 6 months was 1.23 for CaHA and 0.05 for HC. Dramatic differences between CaHA and HC were also noted in Global Aesthetic Improvement Scale (GAIS) ratings at 6 months. For CaHA, 94.6% of folds were graded improved, much improved, or very much improved, compared with 2.7% for HC. Data for up to 3 years has been gathered and is now in review by investigators. Early analysis suggests some residual effect in some patients for up to 36 months (Brian Pilcher, PhD, San Mateo, CA, personal communication, April 2009).

Adverse events were limited to erythema, edema, and ecchymoses. Edema and bruising were more common on the CaHA-treated sides than those treated with HC (*P*<.0001). Edema and bruising lasted approximately 1 week after any injection and the average duration for erythema was approximately 2 to 3 weeks, with no significant difference between the two materials. One nongranulomatous nodule was observed with CaHA compared with three with HC. All adverse events resolved without sequelae. In addition to the CaHA/HC study, another study found longer lasting results and increased satisfaction with CaHA when compared with two hyaluronic acid products.[16]

In a recent study, Busso and colleagues sought to determine whether the addition of anesthetic agents, such as lidocaine, to prefilled CaHA syringes might provide sufficient anesthetic prophylaxis to reduce the need for conventional anesthetic pretreatment procedures. The study demonstrated that the addition of lidocaine to CaHA syringes can be added safely without harmful changes in the physical properties of the original soft-tissue filler.[5] Additional studies are underway to determine whether the addition of lidocaine

alters patients' discomfort, durability, and efficacy. It is the author's opinion that, as described in Busso's manuscript, addition of 0.15 cc 1% lidocaine with epinephrine to the 1.5 cc syringe and mixed by way of a female to female adaptor is revolutionary, dramatically lessens patients' discomfort, and is rapidly becoming the standard of care.

Clinicians have speculated whether CaHA posed any confounding radiographic properties. Carruthers and colleagues set out to answer this question and found that CaHA is not consistently evident on X ray but is clearly visible on CT. However, CaHA is unlikely to be confused with usual abnormal and normal radiographic findings. Although usually visible on CT, its appearance is distinct from surrounding bony structures, does not obscure underlying structures, and does not interfere with normal analysis.[6] In summary, while visible on CT and X ray, CaHA does not interfere with usual interpretation of the radiographs, and therefore, does not pose overt radiographic safety concerns.

Technique
CaHA should be injected in small amounts in a retrograde fashion into the immediate subcutaneous plane or epiperiosteal plane, using a linear retrograde tunneling technique. Cross- hatched linear threading may also be employed. Overcorrection should be avoided. The nondominant index finger should be used to guide the needle and the thumb and forefinger used to mold the product and to remove any contour irregularities. CaHA should be injected very slowly in long, linear microthreads of approximately 0.05 mL per pass. Extreme caution should be taken when injecting into the subdermal plane around the superior nasolabial fold, where the angular artery and branches are present (**Fig. 4**). Occlusion of this vessel can occur by way of external compression from CaHA or by injection of CaHA directly into the lumen of the vessel, creating embolic ischemia

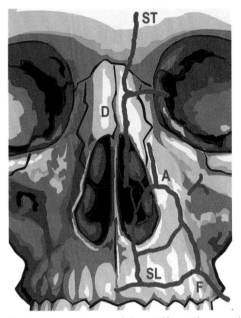

Fig. 4. Vascular anatomy of the midface. The angular artery (a branch of the facial artery) anastomoses with the supratrochlear and dorsal nasal arteries (branches of the ophthalmic artery), joining the external carotid artery network with the internal carotid artery network. Occlusion or embolic events involving this network can lead to extensive tissue necrosis. ST, supratrochlear artery; D, dorsal nasal artery; A, angular artery; SF, superior labial artery; F, facial artery.

and tissue necrosis of the nasal alar region along the distribution of the angular arteries or its branches. Reports of alar vascular necrosis have been reported to the author and the superior nasolabial fold should be considered a high-risk area not only for CaHA but for all injectable fillers.

It is particularly important to use sufficient volume of CaHA for the treatment of HIV-related lipoatrophy. While previous studies have demonstrated different efficacy endpoints, such as photographic documentation of global improvement and change in mean skin thickness using ultrasound or skin calipers, treatment often falls short of optimal correction in clinical practice. In a recent study by Carruthers and Carruthers, the authors defined optimal correction as "very much improved" on the GAIS scale, where a touch up is not required, and sought to determine the volume necessary to achieve optimal correction. Using a mean cumulative volume of 13.4 mL of CaHA, subjects in the Carruthers' study achieved the top GAIS score of "very much improved" in 80% of subjects at 3 months and 59% at 6 months, compared with 26% at 3 months and 7% at 6 months in a similar study by Silvers that used a mean cumulative volume of 8.4 mL of CaHA.[7,8]

Poly-L-lactic Acid

PLA is a synthetic polymer that is biodegradable and resorbable. Injectable PLA (Sculptra, Dermik Laboratories, Berwyn, Pennsylvania) consists of microparticles of PLA in a sodium carboxymethyl-cellulose gel. The filler must be reconstituted with sterile water before administration. No skin test is required. PLA was approved by the FDA in 2004 for the treatment of HIV-related facial lipoatrophy, although the product is used off label for limited age-related lipoatrophy in patients who do not have HIV.

Mechanism of action

PLA is administered into the subcutaneous plane. There, the suspension of reconstituted PLA provides mechanical correction and filling. Immediate volumizing is mostly from fluid that becomes absorbed over a few days. Over weeks to months, the PLA microparticles are gradually degraded, while treated areas undergo subtle volume expansion as the host tissue responds to the PLA.[9] The microparticles of PLA become surrounded in a capsule of connective tissue consisting of connective tissue cells and inflammatory cells, such as macrophages, lymphocytes, mast cells, and foreign body giant cells. As time passes, there is a fibrous-tissue response with collagen deposited around the foreign body reaction. This fibrous response is thought to provide sustained correction.

Indications

PLA is indicated specifically for the correction of HIV-related facial lipoatrophy. It is also approved for correction of nasolabial folds in HIV negative patients. The filler works best for volume correction, not specific depressions. PLA is also used off label in non–HIV-infected patients who have panfacial stage 1 facial lipoatrophy, a condition that is often a consequence of aging in healthy, lean individuals. Monthly injections of one to two vials into the subcutis over many treatments (4–6 is usual) often achieve restoration of subcutaneous volume (**Fig. 5**). Correction of subcutaneous fat loss will often last for 12 to 24 months. After this time, patients will often seek reinjection. In the author's experience, PLA is often not successful in treating more advanced cases of HIV facial lipoatrophy.

Efficacy and safety

PLA was first approved in 2004 using a fast-track process, an accelerated review procedure often used for HIV drugs. Efficacy and safety data for the approval was based on data from physician-sponsored Investigational Device Exemption studies in the United States and the European VEGA study. The VEGA study followed 50 subjects

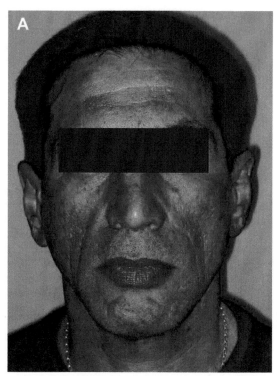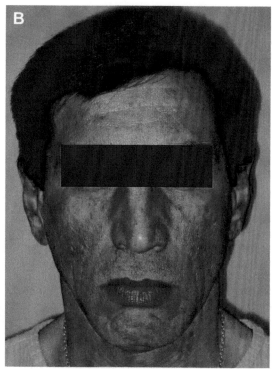

Fig. 5. (*A*) Pretreatment of age-related, non-HIV facial lipoatrophy compared with 1 month following the final treatment with eight vials of Sculptra injected in four treatment sessions over 3 months. (*B*) One month after last injection. (*From* Jones D, Vleggaar D. Technique for injecting poly-L lactic acid. J Drugs Dermatol 2007;6:S13–7; with permission.)

treated with PLA for 96 weeks.[10] Subjects with HIV-associated facial lipoatrophy received four sets of injections: Day 0, followed by every 2 weeks for 6 weeks. Subjects were evaluated using clinical examination, facial ultrasonography, and photography. At entry, the median facial fat thickness was 0 mm. The median total cutaneous thickness increased significantly from baseline (up to 7.2 mm at weeks 48 and 72). By week 96 the median total thickness was 6.8 mm. No significant adverse events were observed. In 22 (44%) subjects, palpable but nonvisible subcutaneous nodules were observed, which tended to spontaneously resolve with time. The study did not use ratings of pre-and posttreatment photographs by experienced physicians not performing the treatment to measure whether optimal correction with complete restoration of cheek contours was achieved. Approval for aesthetic use was gained in mid 2009 based on the results of a randomized, evaluator-blinded, parallel-group, multicenter study of 233 patients carried out in immune competent patients. The treatment phase consisted of 1 to 4 visits at 3-week intervals during which patients received bilateral injections (average of all injections was 2.3 vials) of Sculptra®Aesthetic[11] (n = 116) or collagen (n = 117)

into the left and right nasolabial fold wrinkles. The follow-up phase consisted of visits at week 3 and months 3, 6, 9, and 13 after the last treatment. Of the 116 patients treated with Sculptra®Aesthetic, 106 patients completed the study and continued into the long-term surveillance phase, which extended to 25 months. Ninety-five patients completed the surveillance phase. Evaluation was done through use of the Wrinkle Assessment Score (WAS) coding system, (0 = no wrinkles; 5 = a very deep wrinkle or redundant fold). Improvements from baseline at 25 months proved to be consistent, progressive, and statistically significant at each time point measured (P<0.001) 100% of patients improved at week 3; 88.7% at month 13; and 86.3% at month 25.

Patients consistently reported high satisfaction with their Sculptra®Aesthetic treatment results with 80% of patients satisfied with results at 25 months. In physician-reported adverse events with Sculptra®Aesthetic: 8.6% of patients experienced papules and nodules up to 13 months falling to 1–1.9% at 25 months.

An increased risk of papules and nodules in the periorbital area has been reported in published literature therefore use in the periorbital area is not recommended. Use of Sculptra®Aesthetic is contraindicated in the lips, in individuals with known hypersensitivity to any of its components, or in patients with known history of or susceptibility to keloid formation or hypertrophic scarring. Sculptra®Aesthetic should not be injected in areas with active skin infection or inflammation.

In addition to the adverse events in these studies, persistent granulomatous reactions have been observed (**Fig. 6**).[12]

Technique

PLA should be injected into the subdermal plane, not into the dermis, to limit the likelihood of nodule and papule development. Red, palpable, persistent dermal nodules may occur with intradermal injection. Dermal defects are better treated with an HA or collagen filler. A linear retrograde technique, with a cross-hatching approach, should be used with a 25-gauge, 1-in or 2-in needle. Smaller bore needles tend to become easily clogged. Practitioners should use 1 mL tuberculin syringes, and shake the solution well before transferring to syringe and immediately before injection.

The 25-gauge needle entry site may be anesthetized with small, intradermal injections of 1% lidocaine with epinephrine through a 30-gauge needle, resulting in tolerable injections. Intravascular injection should be avoided; the angular artery runs in the immediate subdermal plane in the area of the superior nasolabial fold. Injection of the parotid duct, which overlies the buccinator muscle in the lateral cheek, should also be avoided.

It is often helpful to outline the treatment area before injection. The treated area must not extend above the inferior orbital rim. To prevent contour irregularity and visible or palpable nodules in the infraorbital area, the product must be injected epiperiosteally in small amounts, deep to the muscle layer, using a serial puncture technique. Patients should also be made aware that the immediate posttreatment appearance will fade within 2 to 4 days. This instantaneous effect is caused by fluid from the filler, which causes edema upon injection. Optimal augmentation will become apparent after multiple treatments at 3- to 4-week intervals, as new collagen is regenerated.[13]

Although the package insert recommends reconstitution of each vial of PLA with 3 mL of sterile water, subcutaneous lumps also can be avoided if each vial is reconstituted with 5 mL of sterile water, or 4 mL of sterile water and 1 mL of 1% lidocaine without epinephrine, at least 24 hours before injection. The reconstituted vial should be vigorously shaken immediately before transfer into the syringe as settling of the product in the syringe may lead to uneven application and contribute to nodule formation.[13] Unlike CaHA, which generally is not massaged by patients, those who have PLA injections should be instructed to frequently massage the treated area in the days to weeks following the procedure to prevent the formation of uneven or lumpy fibroplasia. Some advocate the "rule of 5s" whereby the patient massages the area for 5 minutes, 5 times daily, for 5 days after the injection.

PLA effect is subtle, and many treatments may be required to reach optimal correction. Duration is generally 1 to 2 years.

Hyaluronic Acid Derivatives

Hyaluronic acid, an important natural component of human skin, is a glycosaminoglycan

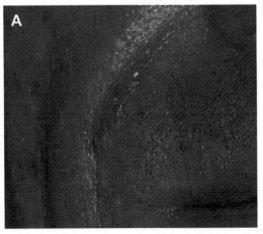
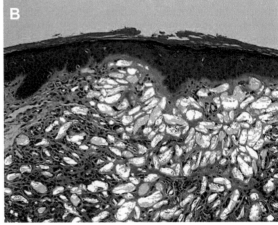

Fig. 6. (*A, B*) Persistent granulomatous reaction to PLA. (*From* Wildemore JK, Jones DH. Persistent granulomatous inflammatory response induced by injectable poly-L-lactic acid for HIV lipoatrophy. Dermatol Surg 2006;32:1407–9; with permission.)

polysaccharide comprised of residues of the monosaccharides d-glucuronic acid and N-acetyl-d-glucosamine. HA fillers comprise the major share of the United States market place for injectable fillers, with Juvederm (Allergan, Irvine, California) and Restylane (Medicis, Scottsdale, Arizona) dominating the market.

Most hyaluronic acid derivatives are superior to bovine collagen 6 months after injection. For example, in the pivotal study comparing three formulations of Juvederm with Zyplast, 81% to 90% of nasolabial folds treated with Juvederm maintained a clinically significant improvement from baseline for at least 6 months, compared with 36% to 45% with bovine collagen.[14] The pivotal trial for Restylane evaluated 138 subjects who received Restylane in one nasolabial fold and Zyplast in the contralateral fold. Using the GAIS, investigators rated 62% of folds superior with Restylane at 6 months compared with Zyplast, and 8% rated Zyplast superior to Restylane.[15]

Generally, hyaluronic acid-derivative–associated correction has a cosmetic effect for approximately twice as long as bovine collagen (ie, persistence for 4–6 months rather than 2–3 months).[6] However, recent studies of nonanimal HA derivatives have demonstrated long-lasting effectiveness of up to 18 months after retreatment with either Juvederm or Restylane because of the apparent development of fibroplasia around the injected product. Therefore, certain hyaluronic acids should be considered semipermanent fillers.[16,17]

Serious adverse events are rare. In a retrospective analysis of the safety of nonanimal, stabilized HA, major adverse events included hypersensitivity reactions, localized granulomatous reactions, bacterial infection, and acneiform and cystic lesions.[18] One salient advantage of hyaluronic acid is that adverse reactions or unwanted placement of product may be quickly and safely reversed with hyaluronidase.[19] Other HA currently FDA-approved include Prevelle Silk (Mentor, Irving, Texas), a 5.5 mg/cc HA with pre-incorporated lidocaine. Compared with Juvederm and Restylane, Prevelle Silk is a less concentrated or lighter HA with less lift capacity and a shorter tissue residence time. Also FDA-approved is Elevess (Anika, Woburn, Massachusetts), which is a higher concentration 28 mg/cc HA (**Table 1**). Several other HA are being investigated in clinical trials in the United States. They include Puragen Plus (Mentor Corporation, Santa Barbara, California), which contains lidocaine integrated directly into the formula; Belotero Soft and Belotero Basic (Anteis, Geneva, Switzerland), and Teosyal (Teoxane Laboratories, Geneva, Switzerland).

PERMANENT FILLERS
Liquid Silicone

Liquid silicone (LIS) was first used as an injectable filler in the 1950s. Before collagen injectable fillers became available in the early 1980s, LIS was the injectable filler of choice. There was no standardized FDA-approved product and many products of varying purity were injected often in large bolus form, which led to frequent product migration and foreign-body reactions. Subsequently, in the early 1990s, all forms of silicone for cosmetic implantation were banned by the FDA because of possible

---

Table 1
Currently available dermal fillers approved by the US Food and Drug Administration (May, 2009)

Temporary fillers	
Bovine collagen	Zyplast, Zyderm (Allergan, Irvine, CA)
Human collagen	Cosmoderm, Cosmoplast (Allergan, Irvine, CA)
Porcine collagen	Evolence (Colbar, Herzliya Israel)
Hyaluronic acid	Prevelle Silk (Mentor, Irving, TX), Elevess (Anika, Woburn, MA)
Semipermanent fillers	
Calcium hydroxylapatite	Radiesse (BioForm, San Mateo, CA)
Poly-L-lactic acid	Sculptra (Dermik, Berwyn, PA)
Hyaluronic acid	Restylane, Perlane (Medicis, Scottsdale, AZ); Juvederm (Allergan, Irvine, CA)
Permanent fillers	
Liquid silicone	Silikon-1000 (Alcon, Fort Worth, TX); Adatosil-5000 (Escalon Ophthalmics, Skillman, NJ)
Polymethyl methacrylate	Artefill (Artes, San Diego, CA)

toxicity and systemic reactions related to LIS and silicone breast implants.

After the FDA resolved safety issues regarding silicone breast implants and LIS, in the late 1990s, two new forms of highly purified liquid silicone were approved (Silikon-1000 and Adatosil-5000) for use as an intraocular implant to treat retinal detachment. While this use is the only official indication for LIS, the FDA Modernization Act of 1997 makes off-label uses legal, provided that the physician or drug manufacturer does not advertise for such use. LIS is now used off label for soft-tissue augmentation (see indications discussed later). Silikon-1000 has a lower viscosity and is the most suitable for injectable soft-tissue augmentation, as it is easier to inject through smaller gauge needles.

Current opinion on liquid injectable silicone is polarized between opponents and advocates. Opponents argue that despite use of proper technique and products, serious adverse events are common and unpredictable. Proponents rely on a wealth of anecdotal data to argue that liquid injectable silicone is safe and effective as long as three rules are employed: (1) use highly purified FDA-approved LIS; (2) employ microdroplet serial puncture technique (defined as 0.01 cc per injection site injected into the subdermal plane); and (3) use small volumes (0.5 mL for smaller defects and up to 2 mL for larger areas of atrophy) at each session with multiple sessions staged at monthly intervals or longer.

Mechanism of action

After LIS is injected, a capsule of new collagen develops to encircle each microdroplet of silicone. This process continues for about 3 months, during which time the collagen capsule adds volume to the augmentation of the LIS microdroplet. The collagen also holds the droplets in place to prevent migration.[9]

Indications

Although LIS is used off label for many indications, it is the author's opinion that LIS should not be routinely employed for the average cosmetic patient until longer-term studies with current products resolve some of the controversy regarding longer-term safety and efficacy. However, for the unique and disfiguring defects associated with HIV facial lipoatrophy and serious acne scarring, LIS produces cosmetically superior and more durable results than currently available less-permanent options (See Efficacy and safety discussed later).

Efficacy and safety

LIS is an excellent choice for HIV-associated facial lipoatrophy. In one trial, highly purified 1000-cSt silicone oil was studied among 77 subjects to determine the number of treatments, amount of silicone, and time required to reach complete correction. Subjects received 2 mL of Silikon 1000 at monthly intervals with the microdroplet technique until optimal correction was achieved. The researchers elucidated two important findings: (1) all three of these parameters were directly related to the initial severity of lipoatrophy, and (2) highly purified 1000-cSt silicon oil is a safe and effective treatment option for HIV-associated lipoatrophy (Fig. 7).[20] Five-year data is now available on this cohort and no serious adverse events have been found (D. Jones, unpublished data).

Using the microdroplet, multiple-injection technique, Barnett and Barnett have had success with injections of LIS for acne scars lasting over a 10-, 15-, and 30-year follow-up periods.[21]

Technique

Clinicians should inject only highly purified FDA-approved LIS, such as Silikon-1000, using the microdroplet serial puncture technique (0.01 mL or less injected through a 27-gauge needle into the immediate subdermal plane at 2 mm to 4 mm intervals). Intradermal injections should be avoided, as these may create intradermal papules.[22] However, intradermal injections may be used for atrophic dermal acne scars, using 0.001 mL microdroplets.

Very small amounts of LIS should be injected at monthly intervals, or longer. The immediate goal is undercorrection. Optimal correction occurs slowly as fibroplasia develops around the microdroplets, creating further tissue augmentation and anchoring each microdroplet into place.

Polymethyl Methacrylate

Injectable PMMA (ArteFill, Artes Medical, San Diego, California) is a suspension of 20% PMMA smooth microspheres and 80% bovine collagen. ArteFill is the product of third-generation PMMA microsphere technology. Previous generations include Arteplast (used in Germany from 1989 to 1994) and Artecoll (used worldwide, except in the United States and Japan, from 1994 to 2006). Artefill represents a third-generation product containing fewer nanoparticles (less than 20 microns), which were thought to be associated with granulomatous reactions observed with previous generations. ArteFill was approved by the FDA in 2006 for the correction of nasolabial folds. However, Artes filed for Chapter 7 bankruptcy in December 2008, and was acquired by

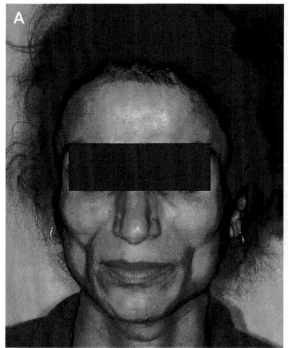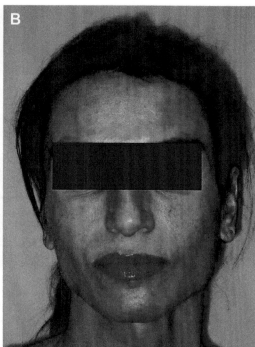

Fig. 7. (*A, B*) Pretreatment and posttreatment liquid injectable silicone for HIV-associated facial lipoatrophy. (*Courtesy of* D. Jones, MD, Los Angeles, CA.)

Suneva (San Diego, California) which now owns and distributes ArteFill.

Mechanism of action

After PMMA is injected, the collagen vehicle is absorbed within 1 to 3 months. Afterward, new collagen is deposited by the host to encapsulate and engulf the remaining estimated 6 million PMMA particles in 1 mL of ArteFill. This process contributes to tissue augmentation through fibroplasia. Although collagen is absorbed, the PMMA is permanent and not reabsorbed.[9]

Indications

Injectable PMMA is indicated for nasolabial folds. It is also used off label for glabellar frown lines, radial lip lines, and mouth corners.

Injectable PMMA is contraindicated for use in patients who have a positive result to the required ArteFill skin test; patients who have severe allergies (as indicated by a history of anaphylaxis or multiple severe allergies); patients who have known lidocaine hypersensitivity; patients who have a history of allergies to bovine collagen products; and patients who have known susceptibility to keloid or hypertrophic scarring. The product should not be used for lip augmentation.

Efficacy and safety

The United States pivotal clinical trial for ArteFill was a controlled, randomized, prospective,

double-masked trial of 251 subjects at eight centers across the United States. Subjects received either ArteFill or bovine collagen dermal filler (control). Efficacy was rated by masked observers using a photographic Facial Fold Assessment Scale. The study demonstrated a significant improvement with Arte-Fill compared with the control group at 6 months ($P<.001$) in nasolabial folds. A subset of subjects was observed at 12 months and all showed persistent wrinkle correction (**Fig. 8**).[23]

A subgroup of 69 subjects returned for follow-up 4 to 5 years later. Investigator Facial Fold Assessment ratings at 4 or 5 years were improved from baseline by 1.67 points ($P<.001$). Nearly all subjects (95.5%) reported that they were at least somewhat satisfied and 81.8% reported that they were either satisfied or very satisfied.[23]

Five subjects reported six late, adverse events that occurred from 2 to 5 years after the initial injection. Of these, four were mild cases of lumpiness, and two were severe. The total number of late, adverse events was 6 of 272 (2.2%) of wrinkles injected.[24]

Granulomatous reactions (manifested by inflamed red nodules) may be treated with intralesional cortisone combined with antibiotic therapy.

Technique

Injectable PMMA is placed into the dermal-subcutaneous junction using the tunneling or linear

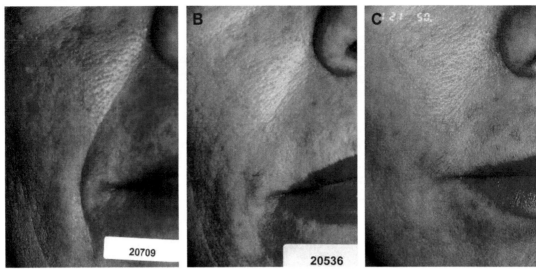

Fig. 8. Results of ArteFill for the treatment of nasolabial folds at pretreatment, 1 year posttreatment, and beyond 1 year posttreatment. (*A*) Pretreatment. (*B*) 1 year posttreatment. (*C*) Greater than 1 year posttreatment. (*From* Cohen SR, Holmes RE. Artecoll: a long-lasting injectable wrinkle filler material: report of a controlled, randomized, multicenter clinical trial of 251 subjects. Plast Reconstr Surg 2004;114:964–76; with permission.)

threading technique with a 26-gauge, 5/8-in needle. Overcorrection is not recommended. It is preferable to inject more deeply than superficially, as the risk of wasted material is less problematic than superficial injection, which can cause permanent skin surface texture or color impairment.

Patients should be evaluated 4 to 6 weeks after the injection to assess the need for further treatments. Optimal correction usually requires two to three treatments, and touch-up implantations should be at intervals of at least 2 weeks or longer depending upon the amount of implant used, the site of placement, and the dynamics of the corrected sites.

Investigational Permanent Agents

Hydrogel polymers

Hydrogel polymers are a novel class of fillers, comprised mostly of water with a small amount of synthetic polymer. The so-called injectable "endoprosthesis" agents include Bio-Alcamid (Polymekon, Milan, Italy) and Aquamid (Aquamid, Ferrosan, Copenhagen, Denmark), both of which are used in Europe but are not yet FDA approved. These nonbiodegradable fillers are composed of 96% water and 4% synthetic polymer (polyalkylimide, in the case of Bio-Alcamid, and polyacrylamide for Aquamid). Both agents are used for large-volume augmentation, such as hemifacial lipoatrophy (Romberg's disease) or HIV-associated lipoatrophy.

Mechanism of action

Once injected, the gel particles become covered by a thin collagen capsule (0.02 mm) which completely surrounds the particles and isolates them from the host tissues, creating an injectable prosthesis. According to the manufacturer, Bio-Alcamid has much stability, integration among living tissues, and more simple removal, if required, than other dermal fillers. The results are considered permanent, but removal can be done through aspiration. Full efficacy of removal through aspiration remains unclear.

Indications

While both agents are used for replacement of facial volume caused by lipoatrophy, they are also used for the treatment of nasolabial folds, lip augmentation, depressed scars, and enhancement of cheekbones and jawline. They are not indicated for the treatment of fine wrinkles.

Efficacy and safety

Recent reports in the literature document the success of Bio-Alcamid for the treatment of HIV-associated facial lipoatrophy.[25,26] According to the manufacturer, risk of infection or allergy is very low (0.6%) and only 0.2% of patients have had an immune response to the implant, which created localized swelling that required drainage over a 1- to 6-month period.

Late-appearing streptococcal bacterial abscesses have been reported. A paper by the author and colleagues follows five patients who received Bio-Alcamid for HIV-associated lipoatrophy and developed late-appearing streptococcal bacterial abscesses (**Fig. 9**).[27] In each case, an acute abscess developed several months and up to years after the initial injection of Bio-Alcamid. All

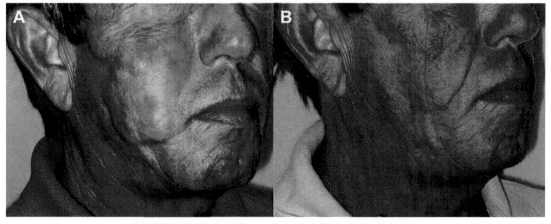

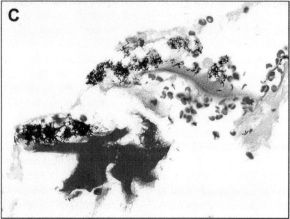

Fig. 9. Bio-Alcamid abscess preincision (*A*) and (*B*) postincision and drainage; gram stain of drained material reveals streptococcal bacteria (*C*). (*Adapted from* Jones DH, Carruthers A, Fitzgerald R, et al. Late-appearing abscesses after injections of nonabsorbable hydrogel polymer for HIV-associated facial lipoatrophy. Dermatol Surg 2007;33:S193–8; with permission.)

five cases responded quickly to drainage and antibiotic therapy, although in two cases the abscesses became recurrent. In one case the patient also developed methicillin-resistant *S. aureus* and required extensive intravenous antibiotic therapy.

Based on the cases, it appears that local oral streptococcal bacteria may be capable of directly invading implant material. It also seems possible that the bacteria may reach the implant through a needle puncture during a dental or surgical procedure, possibly warranting prophylactic antibiotic therapy before dental and surgical procedures in patients who have received Bio-Alcamid.

Bio-Alcamid and other hydrogel polymers carry the risk of foreign-body reaction, infection, migration, or granuloma formation.

Technique

These agents are injected subcutaneously, usually under local anesthesia, and massaged smooth by the clinician. A thin layer of collagen gradually forms around the injected gel over a period of 4 to 8 weeks when the gel becomes completely surrounded and isolated from host tissues, in effect making it an endogenous prosthesis.

SUMMARY

The use of dermal fillers has advanced significantly from its beginnings with fat grafts in the early 20th century to the full array of semipermanent and permanent fillers now available. Today's fillers are suitable for many indications and each has its own advantages and disadvantages.

Many novel dermal fillers that are already available in Europe are now undergoing FDA testing, and some of these will likely be approved for use in the United States within the next few years. They include the aforementioned investigational HA in the semipermanent class of fillers and hydrogel polymers among the permanent fillers. These fillers will expand the choices available to patients and physicians and promise to increase longevity and minimize adverse events.

ACKNOWLEDGMENTS

The author wishes to acknowledge Mark R. Vogel, MA, and David J. Howell, PhD, RRT for their editorial assistance in the preparation of the manuscript.

REFERENCES

1. Klein A, Elson M. The history of substances for soft tissue augmentation. Dermatol Surg 2000;26:1096–105.
2. Coleman KM, Voights R, DeVore DP, et al. Neocollagenesis after injection of calcium hydroxylapatite composition in a canine model. Dermatol Surg 2008;34:S53–5.
3. Berlin AL, Hussain M, Goldberg DJ. Calcium hydroxylapatite filler for facial rejuvenation: a histologic and immunohistochemical analysis. Dermatol Surg 2008;34:S64–7.
4. Smith S, Busso M, McClaren M, et al. A randomized, bilateral, prospective comparison of calcium hydroxylapatite microspheres versus human-based collagen for the correction of nasolabial folds. Dermatol Surg 2007;33:S112–21.
5. Busso M, Voigts R. An investigation of changes in physical properties of injectable calcium hydroxylapatite in a carrier gel when mixed with lidocaine and with lidocaine/epinephrine. Dermatol Surg 2008;34:S16–23.
6. Carruthers A, Liebeskind M, Carruthers J, et al. Radiographic and computed tomographic studies of calcium hydroxylapatite for treatment of HIV-associated facial lipoatrophy and correction of nasolabial folds. Dermatol Surg 2008;34:S78–84.
7. Carruthers A, Carruthers J. Evaluation of injectable calcium hydroxylapatite for the treatment of facial lipoatrophy associated with human immunodeficiency virus. Dermatol Surg 2008;34:1486–99.
8. Silvers SL, Eviatar JA, Eschavez MI, et al. Prospective, open-label, 18-month trial of calcium hydroxylapatite (Radiesse) for facial soft-tissue augmentation in patients with human immunodeficiency virus-associated lipoatrophy: one year durability. Plast Reconstr Surg 2006;118:34S–45S.
9. Alam M, Gladstone H, Kramer E, et al. ASDS guidelines of care: injectable fillers. Dermatol Surg 2008;34:S115–48.
10. Valantin MA, Aubron-Olivier C, Ghosn J, et al. Polylactic acid implants (New-Fill) to correct facial lipoatrophy in HIV-infected patients: results of the open-label study VEGA. AIDS 2003;17:2471–7.
11. Sculptra®Aesthetic Product Information. Dermik Laboratories; 2009.
12. Wildemore JK, Jones DH. Persistent granulomatous inflammatory response induced by injectable poly-L-lactic acid for HIV lipoatrophy. Dermatol Surg 2006;32:1407–9.
13. Jones D, Vleggaar D. Technique for injecting poly-L-lactic acid. J Drugs Dermatol 2007;6:S13–7.
14. Baumann LS, Shamban AT, Lupo MP, et al. Comparison of smooth-gel hyaluronic acid dermal fillers with cross-linked bovine collagen: a multicenter, double-masked randomized, within-subject study. Dermatol Surg 2007;33:S128–35.
15. Narins RS, Brandt F, Leyden J, et al. A randomized, double-blind, multicenter comparison of the efficacy and tolerability of Restylane versus Zyplast for the correction of nasolabial folds. Dermatol Surg 2003; 29:588.
16. Narins RS, Davan SH, Brandt FS, et al. Persistence and improvement of nasolabial fold correction with nonanimal-stabilized hyaluronic acid 100,000 gel particles/mL filler on two treatment schedules: results up to 18 months on two retreatment schedules. Dermatol Surg 2008;34:S2–8.
17. Smith S, Jones D. Efficacy and safety following repeat treatment for a new family of hyaluronic acid based fillers. In: Programs and abstracts of the 64th American Academy of Dermatology Annual Meeting. San Diego (CA), July 26–30, 2006.
18. Lupton JR, Alster TS. Cutaneous hypersensitivity reaction to injectable hyaluronic acid gel. Dermatol Surg 2001;26:135–7.
19. Brody HJ. Use of hyaluronidase in the treatment of granulomatous hyaluronic acid reactions or unwanted hyaluronic acid misplacement. Dermatol Surg 2005;31(8 Pt 1):893–7.
20. Jones D, Carruthers A, Orentreich D, et al. Highly Purified 1000-cST silicon oil for treatment of human immunodeficiency virus-associated facial lipoatrophy: an open pilot trial. Dermatol Surg 2004;30:1279–86.
21. Barnett JG, Barnett GR. Treatment of acne scars with liquid silicone injections: 30-year perspective. Dermatol Surg 2005;31:1542–9.
22. Jones D. HIV facial lipoatrophy: causes and treatment options. Dermatol Surg 2005;31:1519–29.
23. Cohen SR, Holmes RE. Artecoll: a long-lasting injectable wrinkle filler material: report of a controlled, randomized, multicenter clinical trial of 251 subjects. Plast Reconstr Surg 2004;114:964–76.
24. Cohen SR, Berner CF, Busso M, et al. Artefill: a long-lasting injectable wrinkle filler material—summary of the U.S. Food and Drug Administration trials and a progress report on 4- to 5-year outcomes. Plast Reconstr Surg 2006;118(35):64S–76S.
25. Protopapa C, Giuseppe S, Caporale D, et al. Bio-Alcamid in drug-induced lipodystrophy. J Cosmet Laser Ther 2003;5:226–30.
26. Treacy P, Goldberg D. Use of a biopolymer polyalkylimide filler for facial lipodystrophy in HIV-positive patients undergoing treatment with antiretroviral drugs. J Dermatol Surg 2006;32:804–8.
27. Jones DH, Carruthers A, Fitzgerald R, et al. Late-appearing abscesses after injections of nonabsorbable hydrogel polymer for HIV-associated facial lipoatrophy. Dermatol Surg 2007;33:S193–8.

Photorejuvenation

Jill S. Waibel, MD[a,b,c],*

KEYWORDS

- Laser • Vascular laser • Pigmented laser
- Intense pulsed light • Photorejuvenation

Aging is an ongoing process of change, and some of these changes are welcomed. Other changes, however, are less welcome, such as the appearance of wrinkles, brown pigment, or red blood vessels. The aging process depends on a combination of genetic and environmental factors. Each individual has his or her own unique genetic make-up and history of environmental exposures that cause skin to appear older. Aging of skin is accelerated in some cases by genes and disease, but most significantly by the ultraviolet (UV) radiation of the sun.[1] The appearance of aging skin is directly related to the quantitative effects of sun exposure. The UV rays of the sun cause cutaneous changes such as damage to collagen, solar elastosis, telangiectasias, lentigines, rhytid formation; the collective term for these negative effects is photodamage.[2]

Many patients accumulate significant sun exposure through their normal life activities and recreation. Compounding this problem is damage to the environmental systems of the Earth, such as thinning of the ozone layer, that has made the visible signs of aging, skin damage, and dermatologic disease evident in younger individuals.[3] Photodamaged skin is more than wrinkles; it is a mixture of hyperpigmentation, skin laxity, enlarged pores, roughness, wrinkling, and telangiectasia. Photodamage is most severe at the surface of the skin, and is often manifest through red spots, brown spots, excessive wrinkles, and poor skin texture.

Photorejuvenation is the process of using laser and light sources for returning skin to a more youthful appearance.[4] Effective photorejuvenation eliminates wrinkles, brown pigments, and red spots and improves skin texture.

Before lasers, rejuvenation was accomplished through chemical peels, cryosurgery, and dermabrasion.[5,6] However, in the past 2 decades laser and light source technologies have dramatically advanced rejuvenation procedures and produced results far superior to techniques such as chemical peels. Today's patients want not only effective photorejuvenation but also minimal postoperative recovery time, and the nonablative lasers and light sources easily accomplish both.

Three primary types of laser and light sources are deployed to deliver photorejuvenation results with minimal recovery: vascular lasers, pigmented lasers, and intense pulsed light (IPL). All three technologies provide vibrant photorejuvenation that returns skin to a more youthful appearance. In addition to high efficacy, lasers also provide precise depth control, exquisite site targeting, and a safe treatment delivery.[7] Selecting the right laser and light source begins by understanding and balancing a patient's needs and expectations along with their boundaries for postoperative recovery time and acceptance of side-effect profiles.

VASCULAR LASERS
Introduction

The use of lasers in medicine originated to eliminate vascular birthmarks on the skin.[8] There are several laser technologies to treat vascular lesions.

Aging skin often develops dilated small blood vessels (telangiectases), cherry angiomas, and

Financial disclosures: Speaker's bureau Candela, Ellipse, Lumenis.
[a] Private Practice, 7800 S.W. 87th Avenue, Suite, 8200, Miami, FL 33173, USA
[b] Volunteer Dermatology Faculty, Department of Dermatology, Miller School of Medicine, P.O. Box 016250, Miami, FL 33101, USA
[c] Palm Beach Esthetic Dermatology and Laser Center, 1500 North Dixie Highway, Suite 303, West Palm Beach, FL 33401, USA
* Palm Beach Esthetic Dermatology and Laser Center, 1500 North Dixie Highway, Suite 303, West Palm Beach, FL 33401, USA.
E-mail address: jwaibelmd@aol.com

Dermatol Clin 27 (2009) 445–457
doi:10.1016/j.det.2009.08.007
0733-8635/09/$ – see front matter © 2009 Elsevier Inc. All rights reserved.

bruises (senile purpura) (**Fig. 1**). The treatment of facial telangiectasia is one of the most frequent indications for cutaneous laser therapy.[9] Facial telangiectases are amenable to laser treatment, especially via a vascular laser. People with facial erythema and flushing had few options before advances in laser and light therapy, but they are now well served by treatment from a vascular laser.[10]

Telangiectasia of the face occur in at least 10% to 15% of adults and children. Simple telangiectases are small, dilated vessels that are 0.1 to 1.0 mm in diameter.[11] They are commonly located on the midface region and appear as linear red or blue vessels. Exogenous factors can induce or exacerbate telangiectasia. Alcohol, estrogen, corticosteroids, and chronic actinic damage can precipitate their onset.[12] Trauma or postoperative tension resulting from excisions, facelifts, or other plastic surgeries can promote neovascularization, resulting in telangiectases. Telangiectatic vessels are a predominant feature of rosacea, and enlargement of deeper vessels and increased numbers of smaller vessels can manifest as facial erythema and flushing (**Figs. 2** and **3**).

Poikiloderma of Civatte is a clinical condition induced by chronic, excessive sun exposure.[13] It presents as reticulated brown pigmentation and discrete confluent vascular ectasias, hypopigmentation, and prominent telangiectases on the face, neck, and anterior chest region. This is effectively treated with a vascular laser or intense pulse light.

LASER TECHNOLOGY
Historical Perspective

Around 1982, Dr Rox Anderson[14] introduced the theory of selective photothermolysis. The basis of photothermolysis theory is that selective destruction of the target with minimal damage to surrounding structures produces effective treatments and minimizes the risk of postoperative

scarring. Anderson's theory has withstood the test of time and is now the foundation for many state-of-the-art lasers and light sources.

Anderson first applied his theory of photothermolysis to the treatment of port wine stain (PWS). In the late 1970s and early 1980s, the most popular laser for treating PWS was the argon ion laser. Although the argon ion laser was effective in lightening PWS, it often left a scar in the treatment area and the results varied depending on the skills of the operator. To improve treatment efficacy and test his theory, Anderson sought out a new laser design that operated at 577-nm wavelength with a pulse duration of around 1 ms, but no such laser existed.

To research and construct the new laser Anderson worked with a laser manufacturing company, Candela (Wayland, Massachusetts). In the early 1980s, Candela was building pulse dye lasers (PDLs) for specialized research. At Candela, Anderson teamed up with the then Chief Executive Officer, Dr Horace Furumoto, a leading laser scientist specializing in dye lasers.

Working together the 2 men conquered the technical challenges, completed the first PDL, and conducted the first clinical trials in 1985. The PDL delivered effective treatments without scarring the affected area and was used successfully on infants. Candela commercialized the PDL and marketed the first series under the name SPTL-1, for Selective Photothermolysis Laser, after Anderson's theory (James Hsia, personal communication, July 2008).

The PDL has gone through many upgrades and improvements and represents one of the staple tools for effective laser medical and aesthetic patient care. Extending the wavelength from 577 nm to 585 nm and then to 595 nm, which increased the penetration depth of the laser beam, enabled the treatment of bigger vessels and thicker lesions; and higher energies and pulse repetition rates enabled faster treatment times. The addition of

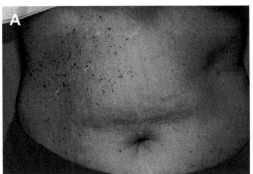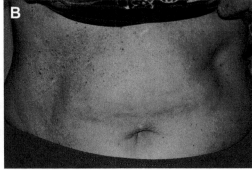

Fig. 1. (*A*) Angiomas baseline 1 month (*B*) after 1 treatment with PDL.

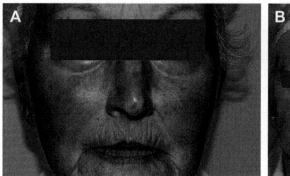
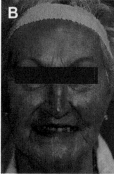

Fig. 2. (A) Facial telangiectasias baseline 1 month (B) after 2 PDL treatments.

a dynamic cooling device (DCD) has reduced treatment discomfort and allowed the safe use of higher treatment fluences for more effective clearance of lesions in fewer treatments. Variable pulse durations have been added for the treatment of various conditions without generating purpura.[15]

The PDL was the first laser to treat vascular lesions, and subsequently many other laser and light systems have been engineered to treat vascular lesions, including potassium titanyl phosphate (KTP), diode, alexandrite, neodymium doped:yttrium-aluminum-garnet (Nd:YAG), and IPL (Table 1).

PDL

The PDL is a versatile tool used for treating a wide variety of conditions, including telangiectasia, rosacea, pigmented lesions, acne, surgical and traumatic scars, skin rejuvenation, leg veins, stretch marks, and wrinkles. The versatility of the PDL often makes it the preferred laser in an aesthetic and medical laser practice. In more than 20 years of clinical use the PDL has built an unprecedented record for safety, mainly because of its close adherence to the principles of selective photothermolysis.

The principal absorbing substance of vascular targets is oxyhemoglobin. The primary absorption peaks of oxyhemoglobin are in the blue-green-yellow portion of the visible range (418, 542, and 577 nm). The longer wavelength penetrates more deeply into the skin with less scattering. By using a laser pulse of about 1 ms in duration, selective damage can be induced in vessels 100 μm in diameter because laser light absorbed by hemoglobin is converted into heat, which damages the endothelium but spares the surrounding connective tissue.[16]

The first-generation PDL had a short-pulse duration of 360 μs. The disadvantage of the shorter-pulsed PDLs is that purpura develops immediately after treatment from extravasation of red blood cells because the laser ruptures the vessel.

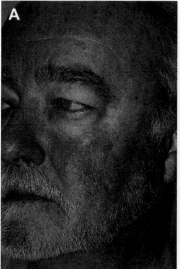
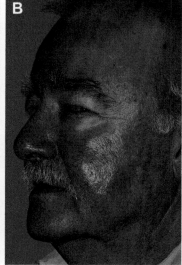

Fig. 3. (A) Rosacea baseline 1 month (B) after 2 PDL treatments.

Table 1
Lasers for vascular lesions

Laser	Wavelength (nm)
Pulsed dye	585, 590, 595, 600
Filtered flashlamp	500–1200
Pulsed KTP	532
Pulsed alexandrite	755
Diode	800
Pulsed Nd:YAG	1064
Pulsed dye and Nd:YAG combined	595, 1064
IPL	550–1200

PDLs with longer pulse durations (10–40 ms) are equally as effective as the original PDL but cause little or no purpura. Longer pulses allow slower heating, less or no vessel rupture, and little or no purpura.[17]

Frequency Nd:YAG Lasers

Several devices exist that emit 532 nm green light at pulse durations of 2 to 50 ms. The 532-nm wavelength is well absorbed by hemoglobin and the longer pulse duration allows for greater and more uniform heating of larger vessels. The KTP laser is a frequency-doubled Nd:YAG that emits green light at 532 nm. The Nd:YAG laser is a solid-state laser containing a crystal rod of YAG doped with neodymium ions. A frequency-doubling crystal made of KTP can be placed in the beam path to emit green light at 532 nm.[18] Advantages of this group of lasers are the absence of postoperative purpura, the result of their longer pulse width that gradually heats the entire vessel without rupturing its walls, and more precise treatment of individual vessels.[19] Immediately after treatment most patients develop mild erythema and swelling, which usually fades within 24 hours.

Diode (800 nm) and Pulsed Alexandrite (755nm) Lasers

Long-pulsed alexandrite (755 nm) and diode lasers (800, 810, and 930 nm) have longer wavelengths within a small peak of hemoglobin absorption for the treatment of deeper, larger vessels. High-powered diode lasers emit energy in the 800-nm region. This longer wavelength penetrates more deeply and is poorly absorbed by melanin, making it safer for patients with darker skin types. Although hemoglobin absorption is less at these wavelengths it is absorbed enough to cause damage to the vessel wall.

Pulsed Nd:YAG (1064 nm) Lasers

Longer wavelengths, such as the Nd:YAG 1064 nm, have the advantage of deeper penetration and poor absorption by melanin. However, because there is a small hemoglobin absorption peak in the 800- to 950-nm range, these lasers still selectively target vascular lesions and veins in particular. Blue reticular veins respond to treatment with the Nd:YAG 1064-nm laser.[20] The Nd:YAG 1064-nm wavelength is not well absorbed by melanin, but is absorbed sufficiently by hemoglobin, making it useful for treating larger, deeper vascular lesions in patients with darker skin types.

Combined Vascular Laser Wavelengths

Combined wavelength lasers are emerging and systems such as 1064 and 595 nm and 532 and 1064 nm are now in clinical use. PDL-heated blood exhibits increased absorption of radiation at 1064 nm, suggesting that the use of combined sequential dual wavelengths may offer benefits compared with single-wavelength treatments. The efficacy of the dual-wavelength laser treatment when compared with Nd:YAG or PDL laser alone was significantly more evident than either single-wavelength treatment ($P<.05$).[21]

IPL Sources

IPL sources deliver light from 515 to 1200 nm at pulse durations ranging from 2 to 25 ms in single, double, or triple pulses. Light is delivered through a rectangular spot size. A coupling gel is applied to the skin before treatment to minimize epidermal damage and increase the efficiency of light delivery to deeper structures. Some IPL devices have cut-off filters that block the transmission of wavelengths below 515, 550, 570, or 590 nm.[22] Some other devices have filter systems that allow transmission of only selected wavelengths, making IPL useful for vascular and pigmented conditions. Advantages of this light source are the absence of postoperative purpura and its wide range of pulse widths that permit treatment of small and large caliber vessels. These devices are also effective for a variety of other vascular and pigmented lesions and for photorejuvenation.

Clinical Applications and Treatment Recommendations

Facial telangiectasia and spider angiomas respond well to 1 or 2 treatments with the PDL, the long-pulsed PDL, the IPL source, or one of the millisecond green pulsed or long-pulsed Nd:YAG lasers. The main drawback to the PDL treatment has been postoperative purpura, which may last 7 to 14 days. The new 3-, 6-, 10-, 20-, and 40-ms PDLs treat these lesions without accompanying purpura, but effective treatment may require multiple or stacked pulses at nonpurpuric intensities. The millisecond green pulsed lasers and the IPL source do not produce any purpura, and multiple treatments may be necessary for complete clearing. Telangiectasias located in the ala nasi and nasolabial groove are more resistant to treatment.

PDLs with variable pulse duration ranging from 0.45 to 40 ms are effective in treating facial ectasias. Improved vessel clearance and reduction of facial erythema can be accomplished with stacking of pulses of lower fluence and longer pulse durations, obviating the need for posttreatment purpura. The mean percentage of vessel clearing following a single treatment improved from 67% with nonoverlapping pulses to 87% with the pulse-stacking technique.[23] It is recommended not to stack more than 4 pulses sequentially.

In addition to eradicating blood vessels, the PDL may also reduce rhytids.

Vascular lasers may improve rhytid improvement and new collagen formation with a 1.5-ms 595-nm PDL. In a study with 595-nm PDLs, Halmi and Roenigk[24] noted with 5 treatments at 4-week intervals a 50% improvement in wrinkles, and a decrease in facial erythema and telangiectasias, and 67% patients noticed tightening of skin and improvement of skin texture. Another study revealed that a 595-nm PDL set at a 0.5-ms pulse width is not an effective means of achieving subpurpuric nonablative periorbital wrinkle reduction.[25]

Preoperatively patients need to have the area cleansed, but patients being treated for telangiectasias and erythema do not require topical anesthesia. Topical anesthesia is discouraged because it causes local vasoconstriction, skin pallor, and lightening of the target chromophore, oxyhemoglobin. By using a large spot size, and a pulse width of at least 6 to 10 ms, the treatment of facial telangiectasia with the PDL may now be effectively performed at subpurpuric fluences. A transient purpura lasting less than several seconds may be seen during the treatment when fluences just below true purpura are used; this is often a good visual clue as to when an appropriate energy setting has been reached. Results may be significantly improved by stacking several nonpurpuric pulses one after another. Stacking should be stopped when the goal of vessel spasm and clearing is achieved, if purpura occurs, or if more than 4 pulses have been delivered. When treating a large area, such as a cheek, pulses may be placed next to each other with a 50% overlap.

This will give the center of treatment area a double pulse and leave the periphery single pulsed and potentially feathered out.

With the KTP and Nd:YAG lasers, the treatment tip is applied along discrete telangiectatic vessels in nonoverlapping pulses. Immediate lightening or disappearance of the target vessel may be observed. Patients are advised that they need not be alarmed if vessels reappear in a few days as these vessels will typically fade away gradually. Retreatment is common and may be repeated at 4-week intervals. A particularly challenging area that may require multiple treatment sessions is the perialar region. Reticular veins are also difficult and require multiple sessions.

Postoperatively, a cool gel pack or packed ice may be applied to the treatment area for palliative relief and temporary swelling. If purpura occurs it usually lasts 7 to 10 days. Mild erythema and swelling can be expected after the treatment of facial telangiectasia or erythema, and typically last 1 to 2 hours post treatment.

Side Effects

When laser treatment is performed with appropriate fluences and proper technique, risks of complications are low. Complications may occur following excessive overlapping of pulses, pulse stacking more than 4 times, excessive energy, or improper patient selection. Scarring (less than 1%), purpura (short term), hyperpigmentation (10%–15%), hypopigmentation (<5%), and infections (extremely rare) were studied with the 585-nm PDL and found to be minimal. There is a higher risk of pigmentary alterations following treatment with the 532-nm lasers. Temporary hyperpigmentation occurs in 25% to 35% of patients and usually resolves in 2 to 3 months. This is more common if patients are exposed to sunlight after laser treatment. Hypopigmentation is uncommon and occurs more frequently in darker skin types (>skin type II) and patients with a suntan. It usually resolves in 3 to 6 months, although it may be permanent. The risk of scarring is low (<1%) and is associated with the use of excessive energies or overlap. There is a higher incidence of scarring in the chest or neck. With proper postoperative care infections are uncommon. However, every patient with a history of herpes simplex virus should be treated prophylactically. A contraindication to treatment is any active infection.

Future Directions

Recent advances in laser technology based on the concept of selective photothermolysis have increased the precision of vascular cutaneous laser surgery. With the introduction of pulsed lasers and light sources photorejuvenation can be achieved effectively and safely. There will be technical developments as more is learned about temperature increases in the skin, new optical imaging devices, and vascular lasers that penetrate even deeper.

PIGMENTED LASERS
Introduction

Aging skin is prone to develop harmless brown lesions. Lasers and IPL sources are frequently used for the cosmetic treatment of pigmented lesions.

Overactivity of the melanocytes may result in blotchy pigmentation. Superficial pigmented lesions, including ephelides, solar lentigines, and flat pigmented seborrheic keratoses, can be effectively treated with most of the pigment-specific lasers (Table 2). Before lasers were available to treat these lesions other destructive methods such as cryosurgery and chemical peels were used, but had side-effect profiles that included scarring, dyspigmentation, skin atrophy, and lesion recurrence.[26] Advances in laser technology have made it possible to remove most benign pigmented epidermal or dermal lesions safely. Because of the cosmetic effect of these lasers and their relative ease of use, they are becoming the mainstay for a variety of pigmented lesions.

Before the lasing of any pigmented lesions a clinical diagnosis should be made. It is advised never to treat any potentially premalignant or malignant lesion with a laser. The treatment of melanocytic nevi is controversial. Goldberg[27] performed a study to evaluate the theoretical concern that laser irradiation may induce malignant transformation of benign nevi. His results in 10 patients showed no significant markers for malignant transformation after Q-switched laser irradiation. Pigment change is the visual marker for malignant melanoma and by removing the nevi malignant transformation may not be recognized.

Laser Technology

The goal when treating cutaneous pigmentation is the selective destruction of undesired pigment with minimal damage to surrounding cutaneous structures. The destruction of pigmented lesions is achieved by the delivery of high energy, at the absorptive wavelength, of the selected chromophore, in this case the melanosome. Current laser therapy targets melanosomes, the melanin-containing organelles contained within melanocytes and keratinocytes. Lasers used to treat melanocytic lesions take advantage of the broad spectrum of melanin ranging from 250 to 1200 nm.[28] The thermal relaxation time of melanosomes is short, ranging from 50 to 500 ns.[29]

Based on the theory of selective photothermolysis, pulse durations on the order of 1 µs or less can selectively damage melanosomes on the order of 1 µ in diameter. Many thermally mediated mechanisms may contribute to the destruction of the melanosome, including thermal denaturation, mechanical damage, and changes in the chemical structure. With high-energy, submicrosecond lasers the rate of local heating and rapid material expansion can lead to structures being torn apart by shock waves, cavitation, or rapid thermal expansion, which shows as immediate whitening or graying of the pigmented lesion. This response correlates with the melanosome rupture seen by electron microscopy. Although the exact cause of the whitening is unknown, it is purported to be the formation of gas bubbles that intensely scatter light. In several minutes these bubbles dissolve, causing the pigmented lesions to return to normal color. Regardless of the cause, immediate whitening offers a clinical compass to an endpoint that most likely represents melansome ruptures.[28] In the ideal clinical situation, only the unwanted pigment is eliminated and the surrounding skin maintains its constitutive pigment. A scab or crust forms that lasts for several days and then the pigmented lesion is exfoliated.[30]

The appropriate selection of devices for the targeted lesion is vital to achieving satisfactory clinical outcomes. Longer-wavelength lasers can penetrate tissue deeper and potentially remove dermal

Table 2	
Lasers for pigmented lesions and dyschromias	
Laser	Wavelength
Long-pulsed lasers	
Long-pulsed alexandrite	755 nm
Long-pulsed ruby	694 nm
Diode laser	800 nm
Long-pulsed Nd:YAG	1064 nm
Long-pulsed dye	595
Q-switched lasers	
Q-switched ruby	694 nm
Q-switched alexandrite	755 nm
Q-switched Nd:YAG	532/1064 nm
IPL	
IPL	515–1200
IPL and RF	

pigment. Shorter-wavelength devices more selectively absorb melanin and may be preferable for more superficial pigmented lesions. Q-switched lasers treat epidermal and dermal pigmented lesions effectively and safely. The 3 Q-switched lasers used for the treatment of superficial epidermal lesions include 532-nm frequency-doubled Q-switched Nd:YAG, the Q-switched 694-nm ruby, and the Q-switched 755-nm alexandrite lasers. The long-pulsed ruby (694-nm) and the long-pulsed alexandrite (755-nm) lasers are well absorbed by melanin and penetrate sufficiently to be effective in the treatment of deeper pigmented lesions. The 1064-nm Nd:YAG laser penetrates very deeply, but is poorly absorbed by melanin, making 532 nm the wavelength of choice when using the Nd:YAG laser to treat epidermal pigmentation. IPL devices are also used to treat pigmented lesions and generalized dyschromia.

The 595-nm PDL recently introduced a new compression handpiece that targets melanin.[31,32] The pigmented convex handpiece directly contacts the skin and this physical compression evacuates blood from the vessel so the melanin does not have a competing chromophore. The laser is fired using 8-micropulse technology with compression to heat up the melanosome. The handpiece is lifted and blood returns to the vessel. The targeted lesions become subtly darker with each pulse and after 2 to 3 minutes there is a ring of erythema around each successfully targeted lentigo.[31] Unlike treatment with the 755-nm alexandrite laser or Q-switched 695-nm ruby laser there is no frosting of the target ephelides.[33]

Recently it has become clear that with slight adjustments the 595-nm third-generation PDL can safely and effectively improve solar lentigines.[34] Solar lentigo can be safely treated, in non-tanned Caucasians and fair-skinned Asians, during the same pass that treats telangiectasias by turning off the DCD and using wide pulse width. Settings recommended by Fisher[34] are: 10 mm spot size, fluence 7.5 to 8.5 J/cm^2, 20 ms pulse duration and no DCD.

Clinical Applications and Treatment Recommendations

One or two laser treatment sessions are usually sufficient to clear most lentigines, although further treatments may be required to treat larger and more resistant lesions (**Figs. 4–7**). Topical anesthesia may or may not be needed when treating pigmented lesions. A topical anesthetic may be placed on the lesion, left to penetrate for 10 to 30 minutes, wiped off and then treatment can be performed. When treating pigmented lesions the laser handpiece should be held perpendicularly to the area to be treated. Pulses should be delivered with 0% to 10% overlap until the entire lesion is treated. Treatment parameters are determined by the type of lesion and the patient's skin type. The desired laser-tissue interaction produces immediate whitening or graying of the treated area with minimal or no epidermal damage or pinpoint bleeding.

If epidermal debris (tissue splatter) is noted the fluence should be lowered. The whitening of the treated area lasts about 15 minutes and an underlying erythematous urticarial reaction may appear around the treated area. In the days following treatment the affected area usually becomes

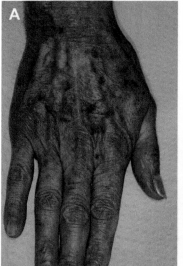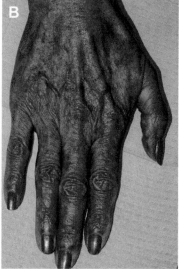

Fig. 4. (A) Solar lentigines baseline 3 months (B) after 1 treatment with alexandrite 755-nm laser.

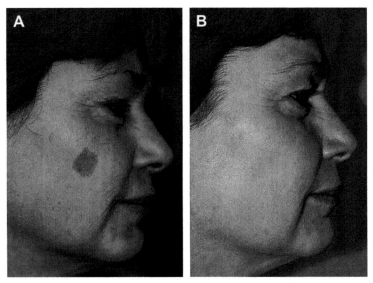

Fig. 5. (A) Solar lentigo baseline 1 month (B) after 1 treatment with alexandrite 755-nm laser.

darker and develops a crust that falls off in 7 to 10 days. Postoperative care consists of application of a healing ointment and avoidance of sun exposure in an effort to reduce the risk of postinflammatory hyperpigmentation. Posttreatment pigmentary changes especially postinflammatory hyperpigmentation are most frequently observed in individuals with skin types III to IV or suntanned skin. Patients with darker skin types should be treated at lower fluences, and pretreatment with topical hydroquinone at least 2 weeks before treatment is advised. Treatment of suntanned individuals should be avoided because of the risk of laser-induced hypopigmentation. Long-pulsed laser and IPL sources are effective for the treatment of lentigines with a low risk of postinflammatory hyperpigmentation.

Side Effects

All medical personnel and the patient must wear the proper protective eyewear to prevent retinal damage. If treating within the orbital rim protective metal ocular shields should be placed over the conjunctiva after a topical anesthetic solution is used to lubricate the eyeshields to minimize the risk of corneal abrasion.[35] Pigment lasers and IPLs are designed to kill pigmented tissue through 3 mm of dermis. Retina and choroid have the most pigment of any place in the body and reside about

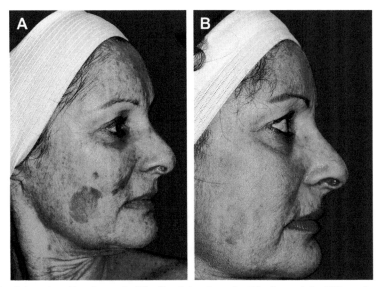

Fig. 6. (A) Solar lentigines baseline 1 month (B) after 1 treatment with alexandrite 755-nm laser.

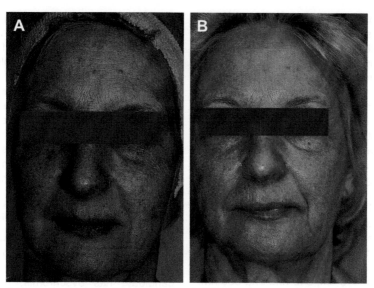

Fig. 7. (A) Periorbital hyperpigmentation baseline 1 month (B) after 1 treatment with alexandrite 755- nm laser.

1 mm deep. Eyelids are on average 2 mm thick, therefore eye injury can occur easily with a laser that targets pigment if it is used without proper safety precautions. If treatment is within the oribital rim, full metal eye shields are recommended. Many topical anesthetics tend to be alkaline and have the potential to burn the cornea. Topical anesthetic agents should not be put under the eyeshields. Topical cooling is often needed to keep the epidermis safe. Cooling may occur in many ways, including DCD, forced air (Zimmer, Ulm, Germany), or mechanical cooling. Cryogen can damage the cornea and it is important to keep the eye protected. Full corneal metal eye shields protect against laser light and cryogen spray. The healing time and the side-effect profile among the pigmented lasers are similar, but infrequent purpura after treatment with Q-switched ruby (694-nm) and alexandrite (755-nm) laser make them slightly preferable to green light, Q-switched Nd:YAG (532-nm) lasers. Pigmentary changes following laser treatment of pigmented lesions are not uncommon. Transient hypopigmentation is most common after treatment with 694-nm or 755-nm wavelengths because absorption by melanin is so strong. Permanent hypopigmentation can be seen with repetitive sessions at higher fluences. Transient hyperpigmentation has also been reported in up to 15% of cases.[36] The incidence of scarring is less than 5% and may be associated with the use of excessive fluences.

Future Directions

Noninvasive real-time optical diagnostic tools are being studied for their role in prelaser diagnosis in pigmented lesions. These tools will also aid in determining in vivo if a lesion has been completely targeted during laser therapy.

IPL
Introduction

Photorejuvenation using IPL is a dynamic, nonablative process defined as a use of noncoherent IPL at a low fluence to rejuvenate the skin. IPLs were first marketed to physicians in the mid 1990s. Since then multiple IPL and combinations of IPL with laser or radiofrequency (RF) sources have become available for nonablative resurfacing. IPL is used to treat a combination of telangiectasias, solar lentigines, and mild rhytids. Because of the wide wavelength spectrum and potential combinations of pulse durations, pulse intervals, and fluences, IPLs have proven to treat efficiently the vascular and pigmented components of photodamage and generalized dyschromia.

IPLs are a mainstay in rejuvenation because of their versatility. IPL fits into a practice with little or no downtime for the treatment of aging skin. IPLs can also rejuvenate many different anatomic locations. When IPL is used for the treatment of epidermal pigment or telangiectasia more sessions are required compared with laser treatment.

Laser Technology

In the past decade photorejuvenation techniques have advanced, allowing significant improvements in the treatment of photoaging. All IPLs use computer-controlled xenon flashlamps and filters to generate light pulses of prescribed duration, intensity, and spectral distribution.[37] Flashlamps are high intensity gas-discharge lamps filled with xenon gas that produce bright light when an electrical current passes through the gas. Newer-generation IPLs have better filtration, improved flashlamps, and added cooling in the handpiece. An IPL can be configured for different emission spectra by varying filtration, lamp type, or current density.[37] Speed is also important, and despite the slow repetition rate (0.3–1 Hz), the large IPL footprints permit rapid treatment of most anatomic areas.[38]

IPL systems are high-intensity polychromatic light sources that emit pulsed light in a broad band of wavelengths between 400 nm and 1200 nm. Cut-off filters are available to narrow the bandwidth of emitted wavelengths to target variable structures selectively at different depths in the skin. Similar to lasers, IPL systems produce their effect based on the principle of selective photothermolysis. The absorption peaks of hemoglobin are approximately 418 nm, 542 nm, and 580 nm, whereas melanin absorbs energy throughout the entire visible spectrum (400–700 nm). Unlike lasers, which treat 1 chromophore with monochromatic light, IPL systems can be used to treat pigmented and vascular lesions simultaneously. There are many IPL systems and they differ in emitted light spectrum (nm), optical filters, fluence, pulse sequence, pulse duration, pulse delay, cooling systems, and spot size. Most systems use some form of protective skin cooling. Early IPL systems had many parameter settings that made it difficult for physicians to find the right combination to optimize therapy. Some newer IPLs have preprogrammed settings based on clinical indications and treated skin types. IPLs are used for treatment of diffuse dyschromia, telangiectasis, pigment, and poikiloderma of Civatte.

There are at least 15 manufacturers and 25 different models of IPL available today. Recent IPL innovations include updated filtering systems, improved pulse generators, and RF and IPL combined for synergy between electrical (RF) and optical energy. Newer-generation IPLs have a dual-mode filter, which limits emissions to the effective wavelengths for more specific targeting. Innovative square-pulse technology maintains energy intensity throughout each pulse.

Clinical Applications and Treatment Recommendations

IPLs are excellent for photorejuvenation of patients with sundamaged skin (**Fig. 8**). The IPL candidate has dyschromia, flushing, rosacea, widespread telangiectasia, need for texture improvement, and enlarged pores. The use of IPLs to eradicate telangiectasia, erythema, and poikiloderma of Civatte (**Fig. 9**) is combined with their ability to destroy lentigines and dyschromia. Improvement in skin texture and mild rhytids is an additional benefit. IPLs and PDLs work well for patients with confluent networks of telangiectasias on the forehead, glabella, nose, cheeks, chin, neck, and upper chest. More recently IPL has been explored for treating mild rhytids. The mechanism of action is thought to be light-induced thermal denaturation of dermal collagen, leading to a reactive cascade of inflammatory mediators and subsequent collagen synthesis. Several studies[39]

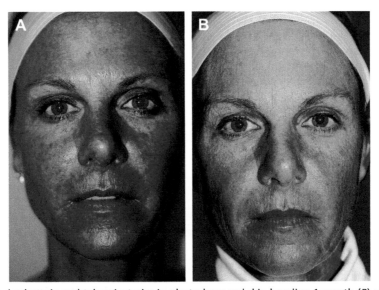

Fig. 8. (*A*) Diffuse dyschromia and telangiectasias in photodamaged skin baseline 1 month (*B*) after 2 treatments with IPL.

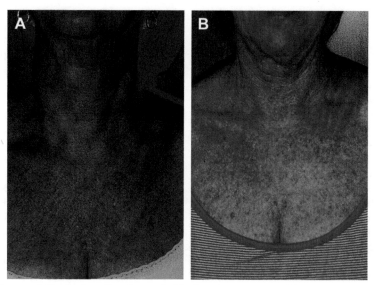

Fig. 9. (*A*) Poikiloderma of Civatte baseline 1 month (*B*) after 1 treatment with IPL.

have shown successful clinical improvement in rhytides after IPL treatment. Nonablative resurfacing with IPL heats dermis to induce collagen coagulation and stimulates fibroblast activity and collagen remodeling. Study of procollagen deposition following IPL treatment in live Yorkshire pig's flank skin revealed significant increase in skin irradiated with procollagen I.[40]

Serial full-face treatments using IPL have been shown to ameliorate the effects of photoaging. Biopsies of photodamaged skin reveal the histologic changes that are typical of sun damage and include atypical keratinocytes, inflammatory infiltrate, telangiectasia, and a zone of altered collagen.[41] After a series of IPL treatments and a biopsy after the fifth treatment, many histologic changes of photodamage were resolved.

The skin is cleansed to remove make-up or any material that may interfere with or absorb the IPL energy. Depending on the device and the patient's pain threshold topical anesthesia may be needed. Appropriate eye protection for all medical personnel present is important. The skin is covered with a layer of cool coupling gel (which should be refrigerated). The handpiece is placed with uniform contact. When the pulse is fired the patient may sense a brief sensation of mild pain and heat. Treatment endpoints are edema and erythema. Treatment endpoints for pigmented lesions include immediate hyperpigmentation.

The IPL is delivered in a series of 5 treatments at 3-week intervals. A broad spectrum of light in the visible and infrared range is used. These treatments help decrease telangiectasia and lentigines. New collagen forms in the skin, which provides

a smoother texture, and fine lines are often decreased. There is little to no downtime after the procedures. Most physicians administer a series of 5 procedures at 2- to 3-week intervals and typically the entire face is treated during each session. Several studies have also shown significant improvement can occur in the neck (poikiloderma of Civatte), the chest (in patients with photodamage) and on the arms and legs.

Side Effects

Newer IPL systems are more user friendly and cause very few major adverse effects; however, if they are used too aggressively scarring can occur. IPL may lead to transient erythema, which usually resolves within hours and can be concealed with make-up. Purpura, dyschromia, blistering, and scarring are rare, with appropriate treatment parameters. For pigmented lesions IPL turns epidermal hyperpigmentation a deepened brown and usually exfoliates within 1 week.

Future Directions

Applications for nonablative resurfacing continue to grow. Additional studies are needed to assess the histologic proof of neocollagenesis with these laser and light devices. Some more recent innovations include combining IPL and bipolar RF. Significant improvement has been made with IPL since the first prototypes: the longevity of the flashlamp has lengthened; rapidness of pulsing has increased; cooling has been integrated into the crystal; and the user interface has been simplified. Tighter filters and new wavelength ranges within heads will continue to propel the IPL technology forward.

SUMMARY

In recent years photorejuvenation techniques have advanced, allowing significant improvements in the treatment of photoaging and vascular and associated pigmentary disorders. The combined use of IPL treatments with other lasers and procedures such as botulinum toxin can simultaneously improve many aspects of cutaneous photoaging. Studies now show the combination of IPL and photodynamic therapy, such as with Levulan, provide new options in the treatment of severely photodamaged skin with IPL. The art of aesthetic dermatologic surgery is achieved by using multiple procedures to solve the complex problems of photoaging skin. Laser photorejuvenation techniques make the reversal of sun-induced damage available to a wide range of patients. The benefits of nonablative procedures are low discomfort, low risk, and minimal postoperative recovery.

REFERENCES

1. Lavker RM. Cutaneous aging: chronological versus photoaging. In: Gilchrest BA, editor. Photodamage. Cambridge (MA): Blackwell Science; 1995. p. 123–35.
2. Taylor CR, Stern RS, Leyden JJ, et al. Photoaging/photodamage and photoprotection. J Am Acad Dermatol 1990;22:1–15.
3. Berneberg M, Plettenberg H, Krutmann J. Photoaging of human skin. Photodermaol Photoimmunol Photomed 2000;16:239–44.
4. Weiss RA, Weiss MA, Beasley KL. Rejuvenation of photoaged skin: 5 years result with intense pulsed light of the face, neck, chest. Dermatol Surg 2002; 28:1115–9.
5. Brody HJ, Monheit GD, Resnick SS, et al. A history of chemical peeling. Dermatol Surg 2000;26:405–9.
6. Lawrence N, Mandy S, Yarborough J, et al. History of dermabrasion. Dermatol Surg 2000;26:95–101.
7. Anderson RR. In: Arndt KA, Dover JS, Olbricht SM, editors. Lasers in cutaneous and aesthetic surgery. Philadelphia: Lippincott-Raven; 1997. p. 25–51.
8. Anderson RR, Parrish JA. Microvasculature can be selectively damaged using dye lasers: a basic theory and experimental evidence in human skin. Lasers Surg Med 1981;1:263–76.
9. Arndt KA. Argon laser therapy of small cutaneous vascular lesions. Arch Dermatol 1982;118:220–4.
10. Lowe NJ, Behr KL, Fitzpatrick R, et al. Flash lamp-pumped dye laser for rosacea-associated telangiectasia and erythema. J Dermatol Surg Oncol 1991;17: 522–5.
11. Kim KH, Rohrer TE, Geronemus RG. Vascular lesions. In: Goldberg DJ, Rohrer TE, Dover JS, et al, editors, Laser and lights, vol. 1. Philadephia: Elsevier Saunders; 2005. p. 11–27.
12. Iyer S, Fitzpatrick RE. Long-pulsed dye laser treatment for facial telangiectasias and erythema. Dermatol Surg 2005;31:898–903.
13. Weiss RA, Goldman MP, Wess MA. Treatment of poikiloderma of Civatte with an intense pulsed light source. Dermatol Surg 2000;26:823–8.
14. Anderson Rox R, Parish JA. Selective photothermolysis: precise microsurgery by selective absorption of pulsed radiation. Science 1983;220:524–6.
15. Kauvar ANB, Lou WW, Zelickson B. Effect of cryogen spray on 595 nm, 1.5 msec pulsed dye laser treatment of port wine stains. Lasers Surg Med 1999;22:19.
16. Dierickx CC, Casparian JM, Venugopalan V, et al. Thermal relaxation time of port wine stain vessels probed in vitro: the need for 1–10 millisecond laser pulse treatment. J Invest Dermatol 1995;105:709–14.
17. Alam M, Dover JS, Arndt KA. Treatment of facial telangiectasia with variable-pulse high fluence pulsed-dye laser: comparison of efficacy with fluences immediately above and below pupura threshold. Dermatol Surg 2003;29(7):681–4.
18. Lanigan SW. Laser treatment of vascular lesions. In: Goldberg DJ, editor. Laser dermatology. New York: Springer Berlin Heidelberg; 2005. p. 13–34.
19. Pence B, Aybey B, Ergenekon G. Outcomes of 532 nm frequency-doubled Nd:YAG laser use in the treatment of port wine stains. Dermatol Surg 2005; 31:509–17.
20. Eremia S, Li CY. Treatment of facial veins with a cryogen spray variable pulse width 1064 Nd:YAG laser: a prospective study of 17 patients. Dermatol Surg 2002:28:244–247.
21. Syrus K, Roos S, Raulin C. Treatment of facial telangiectasia using a dual-wavelength laser system (595 and 1,064 nm): a randomized controlled trial with blinded response evaluation. Dermatol Surg 2008; 34(5):702–8.
22. Schroeter CA, Neumann HAM. An intense light source. The photoderm VL-flashlamp as a new treatment possibility for vascular lesions. Dermatol Surg 1998;24:743–8.
23. Rohrer TE, Chatrah V, Iyengar V. Does pulse stacking improve the results of treatment with variable-pulse pulsed dye lasers? Dermatol Surg 2004;30: 163–7.
24. Halmi BH, Roenigk HH. Using a 595 nm and a 585 nm PDL at a pulse duration of 0.5 msec for periorbital rhytids. Surg Lasers Med abstracts 2004; 30(S14):58–87.
25. Reynolds N, Thomas K, Baker L, et al. Pulsed dye laser and non-ablative wrinkle reduction. Lasers Surg Med 2004;34(2):109–13.

26. Alster TS, Lupton JR. Laser therapy for cutaneous hyperpigmentation and pigmented lesions. Dermatol Ther 2001;14:46–54.

27. Goldberg, D. Laser treatment of Nevi. Program and abstract of American Surgery Lasers and Medicine Society, 2006.

28. Dierickx CC. Laser treatment of pigmented lesions. In: Goldberg DJ, editor. Laser dermatology. New York: Springer Berlin Heidelberg; 2004. p. 37–59.

29. Kilmer SL, Alster TS. Laser treatment of tattoos and pigmented lesions. Cosmetic Laser Surgery 1996;111–28.

30. Dover JS, Geronemus MD, Arndt KA, et al. Pulsed lasers for pigmented lesions. In: Medina M, Shephard C, Phillips M, editors. Illustrated cutaneous & aesthetic laser surgery. Stamford (CT): Appleton & Lange; 2000. p. 241–63.

31. Garden JM, Bakus AD, Domankevitz Y. Cutaneous compression for the laser treatment of epidermal pigmented lesions with the 595 nm pulsed dye laser. Dermatol Surg 2008;34:179–83.

32. Galeckas KJ, Collins M, Ross EV, et al. Split-face treatment of facial dyschromia: pulsed dye laser with a compression handpiece versus intense pulsed light. Dermatol Surg 2008;34:672–89.

33. Kauvar ANB, Rosen N, Khrom T. A newly modified 595 nm pulsed dye laser with compression handpiece for the treatment of photodamaged skin. Lasers Surg Med 2006;38:808–13.

34. Fisher G. Vbeam treatment for skin rejuvenation. Candela Clinical Bulletin 2008. Available at: www.candelalaser.com.

35. Hammes S, Augustin A, Raulin, et al. Pupil damage after periorbital laser treatment of a port-wine stain. Arch Dermatol 2007;143(3):392–4.

36. Kilmer SI, Casparian JM, Wimberely JM, et al. Hazards of Q-switched lasers. Lasers Surg Med 1993;S5:56.

37. Ross EV. Laser vs. intense pulsed light: competing technologies in dermatology. Lasers Surg Med 2006:38:261–272.

38. Ross EV, Smirnov M, Pankratov M, et al. Intense pulsed light and laser treatment of facial telangiectasias and dyspigmentation: some theoretical and practical comparisons. Dermatol Surg 2005; 31(9 pt 2):1188–98.

39. Goldberg D. New collagen formation after dermal remodeling with an intense pulsed light in the treatment of photoaging. J Cutan Laser Ther 2002;2:59–61.

40. Iyer S, Carranza D, Kolodney M, et al. Evaluation of procollagen I deposition after intense pulsed light treatments at varying parameters in a porcine model. J Cosmet Laser Ther 2007;9(2):75–8.

41. Bitter PH. Noninvasive rejuvenation of photodamaged skin using serial, full-face intense pulsed light treatments. Dermatol Surg 2000;26:835–42.

Multimodal Treatment of Acne, Acne Scars and Pigmentation

Ava T. Shamban, MD, FAAD[a],*, Vic A. Narurkar, MD, FAAD[b]

KEYWORDS

- Acne • Acne grading scale • Inflammatory acne
- Mulitmodal treatment • Photopneumatic
- Pigmentation • Scarring

Acne is a common skin disease that affects nearly 80% of adolescents and young adults aged 11 to 30 years.[1–4] Acne can present at any age, affecting 8% of adults aged 25 to 34 years and 3% of those aged 35 to 44 years.[4,5] Lesions appear primarily on the face, back, chest, and other areas with a high concentration of pilosebaceous glands.[6]

The development of inflammatory lesions often drives acne patients to seek treatment. If a lesion becomes severely inflamed it may leave a scar. (Scarring may also result in less severe cases of acne.)[6] Severe scarring caused by acne is associated with substantial physical and psychological distress, particularly in adolescents. Scarring may be permanent on the chest and back and on the face. Acne scars affect males and females of all ethnic backgrounds and facial scarring may occur in up to 95% of acne patients.[4]

The pilosebaceous unit (PSU) is the site at which acne originates on the skin. The PSU consists of sebaceous glands, a hair follicle with a canal lined with stratified squamous epithelial cells, and a rudimentary hair shaft. PSU growth and differentiation depend on androgens, growth factors, thyroid hormones, and other biologic factors.[4,7]

Sebum must be produced for acne to develop. Secreted by sebaceous glands, sebum consists of fatty acids that support colonization by *Propionibacterium acnes*, the bacterium associated with acne. Sebum production is increased by androgens and suppressed by isotretinoin.[8]

In normal skin, cells die and are replaced, and sebum sweeps desquamated epithelial cells up the follicular canal and toward the infundibulum, an opening at the top of the follicle. If the infundibulum becomes occluded, as in acne, sebum and dequamated cells accumulate in the canal, forming a medium for the growth of bacteria, triggering immune reactions and inflammation.[4,7]

In summary, 4 major factors contribute to the development of acne: (1) sebaceous gland hyperplasia and seborrhea; (2) altered growth and differentiation of hair follicular cells; (3) proliferation of *P acnes* in the affected follicle; and (4) inflammation with an immune response.[6] Sebaceous hyperplasia and altered follicular growth and differentiation together induce the development of microcomedones, the microscopic precursor to all acne lesions. The inflammatory cytokine interleukin 1α (IL-1α) may also be involved, as it has been shown to induce hyperkeratinization in vitro.[9,10] A microcomedone can become a noninflammatory comedo or, if it becomes inflamed, a pustule, papule, or nodule.[6,7,11]

THE ROLE OF ANDROGENS

In acne-prone children aged 7 to 8 years, androgens stimulate the sebaceous glands to enlarge, increasing (1) the number of lobules per gland, (2) the size of the sebaceous follicle, and (3) sebum secretion. The result is a microcomedo. Sebocyte differentiation is initiated when circulating androgens enter the cell and couple with the androgen receptor, which in turn initiates gene transcription and sebocyte differentiation and maturation. As

[a] Laser Institute for Derm and European Skin Care, #600-E, 2021 Santa Monica Boulevard, Santa Monica, CA 90404-2208, USA
[b] Ste 505, 2100 Webster Street, San Francisco, CA 94115-2381, USA
* Corresponding author.
E-mail address: avasham@aol.com (A.T. Shamban).

Dermatol Clin 27 (2009) 459–471
doi:10.1016/j.det.2009.08.010
0733-8635/09/$ – see front matter © 2009 Elsevier Inc. All rights reserved.

differentiation progresses, the sebocyte ruptures and releases lipids into the sebaceous duct and follicle. At this sebhorrheic stage the follicle is ready for the development of a microcomedo.

Although androgens are stimulating sebocyte differentiation, keratinocytes in the hair follicle are hyperproliferating and accumulating rather than being shed as single cells into the lumen. They become densely packed among lipid droplets and monofilaments. As lipids, bacteria, and cell fragments accumulate in the hair follicle, comedogenesis occurs and an acne lesion appears on the skin.[6,7]

Although androgens play a role in acne, endocrine abnormalities are not detected in most acne patients[6,7,12] and a relationship between severity of acne and levels of circulating andogens has not been proven.[13] Endocrinologic testing in patients with acne is recommended only when evidence of hypergonadism is present.[12]

P ACNES

The microenvironment of the follicle is believed to be important in the pathogenesis of acne because it encourages the proliferation of P acnes into the follicular duct, resulting in an inflammatory papule or pustule. P acnes is a Gram-positive anaerobe whose role in acne is thought to be inflammatory rather than infectious. P acnes induces monocytes to produce tumor necrosis factor α (TNF-α), IL-1β, IL-8, and other proinflammatory cytokines by a mechanism thought to involve pattern recognition receptors such as the recently described toll-like receptors.[10] IL-8 and other chemotactic factors may also be important in attracting neutrophils to the PSU. P acnes also produces proteases, hyaluronidases, and lipases that contribute to tissue injury.[10]

Although the exact way in which P acnes colonizes the follicular duct is not known, reduction in P acnes is correlated with clinical improvement in acne. P acnes reduction is also associated with decreases in proinflammatory mediators.

INFLAMMATION

Severity of inflammation is associated with interactions between P acnes cells, antibodies, complement, and immune responses. CD4 lymphocytes and later, neutrophils, migrate to the follicular wall where they cause disruption, releasing corneocytes, lipids, and bacteria into the surrounding dermis. When this occurs, more inflammatory cytokines are recruited to the scene.[6,7,10] Recent evidence shows that sebocytes express neuropeptides, including substance P, which contributes to abnormal sebocyte differentiation, proliferation, and lipid synthesis.[6]

CLINICAL PRESENTATION

Patients with acne present with varying degrees of disease severity. Acne grading systems have been based on estimates of the types and number of lesions, the most frequently occurring lesion, and anatomic areas of involvement.[14] Comedones may be open (blackheads) or closed (whiteheads). Open comedones, which consist of sebum and desquamated keratinous cells and have a dilated opening, are slightly elevated or flat lesions 1 to 5 mm in diameter. They may resolve without treatment or become inflamed.[4] Closed comedones, which develop as follicles become occluded and sebum accumulates, present as firm, pale, slightly raised lesions 1 to 2 mm in diameter. Microcysts, or closed macrocomedones, may grow to 5 mm diameter. If the follicular sac of a closed comedone ruptures and discharges its contents into the upper layers of skin, an elevated, pus-containing lesion (pustule) develops, which may resolve without scarring. If the sebum and desquamated cells are released into the deeper dermal layers, raised solid lesions, or papules, develop, which require more time to resolve, and scarring often occurs. Nodules, which may become 10 mm in diameter, are deep-seated abscesses that occur in the most severe cases of acne.[4]

TREATMENT OF ACNE

The goals in treating acne are to relieve clinical symptoms and to prevent scarring. Since the extent and type of scarring are associated with the severity and longevity of acne before therapy is initiated[4]), dermatologists encourage patients to obtain early treatment.[8]

Treatment of acne should be aimed at the pathogenic causes and clinical symptoms. The following therapeutic goals have been recommended[4]:

1. reduce production of sebum
2. reverse hyperproliferation and normalize keratinization
3. resolve microcomedones and comedones
4. reduce colonization of P acnes and inflammation
5. prevent formation of microcomedones, comedones, and inflammatory lesions
6. resolve existing inflammatory lesions

An expert comittee[7] has recently updated the 2003 Evidence-Based Consensus Guidelines[6] of the Global Alliance to Improve Outcomes for the Treatment of Acne. The update is based on the greater understanding of acne pathogenesis since the guidelines were published.

The recommendation is to combine treatments to target the maximum number of pathogenic factors.[7]

More specifically, the authors of the 2006 update recommend that clinicians:

- use a topical retinoid as the foundation of treatment for most acne patients because retinoids target the microcomedo, comedones, and inflammation;
- combine topical retinoids with antimicrobial agents;
- use oral antibiotics only in moderate-to-severe acne, not as monotherapy, and discontinue as soon as possible; and
- use topical retinoids as an important part of maintenance therapy

The most important change from the 2003 guidelines is the central role of topical retinoids in the therapy of most acne patients. Other recommendations are that topical retinoids should be used as monotherapy when comedones predominate or in combination with antimicrobial medications, depending on the amount of inflammation; hormones with oral contraceptive agents may be appropriate for female patients; and oral isotretinoin is appropriate for patients with severe acne or in patients who fail topical retinoids, benzoyl peroxide (BPO), or oral antibiotic agents.[7]

One year later (2008) Strauss and colleagues[12] reported guidelines for managing acne vulgaris (but not scarring, postinflammatory erythema, or postinflammatory hyperpigmentation [PIH]) in adolescents and adults. (Laser and light therapies were not included.) The guidelines were developed according to the American Academy of Dermatology (AAD)/American Academy of Dermatology Association "Administrative Regulations for Evidence-Based Clinical Practice Guidelines." All AAD members had the opportunity to review and comment, and the guidelines were subject to final review by the AAD Board of Directors. The content of this report is summarized in this article.

Topical therapy is considered the standard of care. Because retinoids reduce follicular obstruction, they are important topical agents in the treatment of comedonal and inflammatory acne. Skin irritation with current retinoid formulations may require substitution of the less potent salicylic acid. BPO is effective, but a consensus for relative efficacies of different formulations is not available. Since BPO can prevent or eliminate resistance of P acnes to oral or topical antibiotics, it is often used in combination with these agents. Erythromycin and clindamycin are effective and well tolerated but bacterial resistance may limit their use as monotherapies. Azelaic acid appears to be effective against comedones and bacteria in acne.

Combinations of topical retinoids and topical clindamycin or erythromycin are more effective than any of these agents alone. Efficacy improves when either of these antibiotics is combined with BPO.

Systemic antibiotics are standard for managing moderate-to-severe acne and inflammatory acne refractory to other treatments. Minocycline and doxycycline are considered more effective than tetracycline. Bacterial resistance has been reported with all antibiotics but is most common with erythromycin. Use of erythromycin should be limited to patients in whom tetracyclines are contraindicated (pregnant women, children less than 8 years of age). Since bacterial resistance has been increasing, the authors recommend not treating less severe acne with oral antibiotics and, when it is necessary to use them, discontinuing their use as quickly as possible. Trimethoprin, sulfamethoxazole, or their combination are alternatives when other antibiotics cannot be used. Adverse effects associated with systemic antibiotic use include vaginal candidiasis, photosensitivity (doxycycline), and pigment deposition in skin, mucous membranes, and teeth (minocycline). The incidence of such adverse effects is low.

Hormonal agents include oral contraceptives, spironolactone (oral), cyproterone acetate, and oral corticosteroids. Estrogen-containing contraceptives for the treatment of acne in women are supported by clinical trial data. At high doses the antiandrogen spironolactone is effective against acne by blocking androgen receptors. It may also cause hyperkalemia or menstrual irregularity. Cyproterone in combination with ethinyl estradiol (as oral contraceptive) is effective in women, particularly at high doses. The combination of cyproterone and estrogen-containing oral contraceptives is not approved for use in the United States. Brief courses of high-dose oral corticosteroids may be effective against highly inflammatory acne.

Oral isotretinoin is approved for the treatment of severe recalcitrant nodular acne. It is also considered useful in managing acne that is less severe and resists treatment or acne that causes psychological or physical scars. Its teratogenicity and incidence of mood disorders, depression, and suicide (although a cause-and-effect relationship has not been shown) mandates that patients taking the drug register and adhere to the iPLEDGE program.[12]

Intralesional injection of corticosteroids has been shown to improve lesions of cystic acne. Removing comedones, although it does not affect the course of acne, improves the patient's appearance. Herbal and alternative therapies have little supportive safety and efficacy data, although topical tea tree oil was shown to be effective in one clinical trial. Evidence of a role of diet in acne has not been reported at the time of this writing.

The results of clinical trials of topical tretinoin, adapalene, and tazarotene were summarized in a 2006 report.[7] All 3 agents reduce the formation of microcomedones and are approved for use in the United States. Tretinoin reduces comedones and inflammatory lesions and is available in a variety of formulations and strengths. Two formulations, tretinoin microsphere and polymerized tretinoin, were developed to address skin irritation in the original preparations.

Adalapene, a naphthoic acid derivative with retinoic activity, was designed to penetrate the PSU and is tolerated better than any retinoid studied so far. The efficacy of adalapene is comparable to that of tretinoin and is stable when used in combination with BPO. When compared with tretinoin cream, tazarotene may be more effective against papules and open comedones and equally as effective against closed comedones.

Combining therapeutic agents to target different pathologic factors in acne results in increased efficacy, more rapid resolution of lesions, and reduced likelihood of antibiotic resistance.[7] For example, a topical retinoid in combination with either an antibiotic (oral or topical) or BPO is the standard of care for inflammatory or comedonal acne. The retinoid acts against comedogenesis and inflammation and the antibiotic reduces the proliferation of *P acnes*.[4] Since Mills and Kligman[15] showed that topical tretinoin solution combined with erythromycin solution was more effective against moderately severe acne than tretinoin, erythromycin, or vehicle alone, subsequent reports have shown that a variety of other topical combinations (tretinoin and clindamycin or erythromycin, adapalene and clindamycin, doxycycline, or lymecycline) more effective than the antibiotic monotherapies.[4,7] Other advantages are that retinoids probably enhance penetration of antimicrobial agents through the skin[6] and the quick and longer-lasting effects of combinations probably improve compliance and psychological well-being[7] Combining oral and topical antibiotics is not recommended because it provides no additional benefit and may increase the risk of bacterial resistance.[11]

LASER AND LIGHT-BASED THERAPIES

Physical methods for the treatment of acne, including laser and light-based procedures, have been reviewed in detail by Taub.[16] Laser and light-based therapies target *P acnes*, the sebaceous gland, or the infundibulum of the hair follicle.[17]

The effectiveness of visible light in the treatment of acne is caused primarily by the photosensitivity of porphyrins produced by *P acnes*. Upon irradiation with absorbed wavelengths, porphyrins produce reactive, cytotoxic free radicals and singlet oxygen.[17] Protoporphyrin IX, for example, has absorption peaks at 410, 505, 540, 580, and 630 nm. Although maximum absorption occurs at 410 nm (blue), penetration of this wavelength into the skin is less than at the longer wavelength peaks. For this reason, selection of wavelength for the treatment of acne must be a trade-off between absorption efficiency and penetration depth.[16]

A landmark study of the use of phototherapy for the treatment of mild-to-moderate acne was reported by Papageorgiou and colleagues in 2000.[18] In this study, 107 patients were randomized to 4 treatment groups: blue light, blue and red light, cool white light, and BPO cream. Patients were treated once daily for 12 weeks. At the end of the study period, the most improvement in inflammatory lesions (76%) and comedones (58%) was observed with the mixture of blue and red light. The authors attributed this observation to the antibacterial effects of blue light and the probable antiinflammatory effects of red light. Efficacies of blue light and BPO cream were similar and cool white light was the least effective. Adverse effects were not clinically significant in any of the 4 treatment groups.

The report of Papageorgiou and colleagues was followed by a series of reports of the efficacy and safety of devices using blue light at 405 to 420 nm[19–21] and 400 to 440 nm,[22] pulsed light at 430 to 1100 nm,[23] blue light light-emitting diode (LED) at 409 to 419 nm[24] and 415 nm,[25] and 415-nm blue light and 633-nm red light LED.[26] Gold and colleagues (2005)[27] reported the first study to compare blue light with clindamycin, a well-known topical antibiotic agent. A major limitation of these studies is that clinical benefits beyond 2 to 4 months were not addressed.[16]

Light-based therapies for acne are costly, require multiple treatment sessions, and may not be covered by insurance companies.[16] They do not require ongoing patient compliance as do topical and oral agents and may succeed in patients who have failed conventional therapy.[28]

Various laser-based therapies for acne have been studied. A major advantage of laser devices is that wavelength, pulse duration, and fluence can be adjusted to treat specific lesions.[29]

A 1999 study on the use of the pulsed-dye laser (PDL) showed that treatment reduced the size of the sebaceous glands in patients with sebaceous gland hyperplasia.[30] Four years later Seaton and colleagues[31] reported the first randomized double blind controlled trial of the 585-nm PDL in the treatment of mild-to-moderate facial acne. After a single treatment, total lesion counts were reduced by 53% compared with 9% in controls. Pain during treatment and transient purpura, dry skin, and dry lips were also noted. In contrast, Orringer and colleagues,[32] in their randomized split-faced controlled trial, found no significant difference in lesion counts or graded severity between patients treated twice with a 585-nm PDL and placebo. Adverse effects included bruising, hyperpigmentation, erythema, and cyanosis. The reasons for the contrasting results are not clear.[16]

An early study[33] of the effects of 1450-nm laser energy showed that treatment was associated with necrosis of the sebaceous gland that correlated with clinical reduction in truncal acne lesions for up to 24 weeks after the final of 4 treatments spaced 3 weeks apart. These encouraging results stimulated further evaluation of the 1450-nm diode laser by 3 other groups.[34–36] After 3 treatments of 19 patients with mild-to-severe inflammatory facial acne, Friedman and colleagues[34] reported progressively greater reductions in lesion counts after 1 (37%), 2 (58%), and 3 (83) treatment sessions. Patients used topical and oral medications during the study period. Pain during treatment and transient edema and erythema were noted. Jih and colleagues,[35] in their randomized, split-faced, dose-response study of 20 patients with inflammatory facial acne, reported 76% and 70% mean lesion count reductions with only transient erythema and edema at 12 months after 3 treatments at 2 different fluences. Wang and colleagues[36] reported a randomized, controlled, split-faced study in which they obtained a 56% reduction in lesion counts after 4 laser treatments with transient adverse effects.

Used primarily to treat vascular lesions, the potassium titanyl phosphate (KTP) laser is believed to activate bacterial porphyrins and possibly cause thermal injury to sebaceous glands because it penetrates 1 to 2 mm into the dermis.[17] In 2003 Lee[37] presented a study in which 25 patients were treated with the KTP laser alone, 25 were treated with the laser and then with topical medications, and 125 were treated with the laser and topical agents at the same time. Patients were followed for up to 24 months. After 6 laser treatments, laser-only patients achieved 60% to 70% clearance; the other two groups achieved 80% to 95% improvement. Half of the 125 patients maintained clinical benefit for 4 months without additional treatment. The 2 groups receiving topical agents had fewer flares, greater clearance, and faster response times than the laser-only group. Although no patients were treated only with topical medications, the results of this study suggest that lasers provide a benefit comparable to that of oral antibiotics when used in combination with topical agents.[17] The results also highlight the benefit of combination therapies for acne.

The KTP laser has been evaluated by Baugh and Kucaba[38] in 26 patients with mild to moderate facial acne. After 4 treatment sessions, these investigators reported 35% and 21% reduction in acne scores at 1 week and 4 weeks, respectively. Clinical results were supported by histologic data that showed a wound-healing response. Adverse effects were not reported.

Glaich and colleagues[39] treated 15 patients (with mild to moderate facial acne) 3 times with a sequential combination of a 595-nm PDL and a 1450-nm diode laser. As in the study of Friedman and colleagues,[34] lesion counts were progressively reduced after 1 (52%), 2 (63%), and 3 (84%) treatments, and patients continued to use topical and oral antiacne medications during the study period. Adverse effects were limited to mild transient edema and erythema. Photopneumatic therapy, a new modality that combines the delivery of light with pneumatic energy, will be discussed in detail in a later section on acne grading scales.

PHOTODYNAMIC THERAPY

Photodynamic therapy (PDT) for the treatment of acne vulgaris has been reviewed in detail by several groups.[16,40–43] The photodynamic process involves photosensitizing agents that accumulate in the tissue of interest and can be activated by light in the presence of oxygen to produce unstable intermediates that destroy the cells in which they are produced.[42] Kennedy and colleagues[44] introduced a topical formulation of aminolevulinic acid (ALA) that could penetrate the stratum corneum of actinically damaged cells, basal and squamous cell carcinomas, solar keratoses, and pilosebaceous units. ALA is a natural precursor of photosensitive protoporphyrin IX (PpIX) in heme biosynthesis. When sufficient ALA has entered the epidermis and been converted to PpIX, the treated area is irradiated with light that includes wavelengths absorbed by PpIX. The ALA-induced PpIX is converted (in the presence of oxygen) to cytotoxic intermediates. Two photosensitizing agents, ALA and methyl aminolevulinate (MAL), have been studied extensively for the treatment of acne vulgaris. MAL (Metvix, PhotoCure ASA, Oslo, Norway) is a lipophilic ALA derivative designed to penetrate cells more rapidly than ALA. Once in the epidermis, MAL would be enzymatically hydrolyzed to ALA for subsequent conversion to PpIX.[42]

The initial studies of Divaris and colleagues,[45] who demonstrated the presence of PpIX in sebaceous glands of mice injected intraperitoneally with ALA, and Hongcharu and colleagues,[46] who reported decreases in sebum excretion rates, suppression of bacterial porphyrin fluorescence in sebaceous follicles, and damaged sebaceous glands after ALA PDT, launched a series of reports describing the use of various laser or light sources in PDT for mild to severe acne.[16,41–43] In a 2006 consensus report,[42] panel members agreed that "ALA PDT provides (1) the best results when used to treat inflammatory and cystic acne and (2) modest clearance when used to treat comedonal acne," although recent data shows that ALA PDT was effective against comedonal acne[47] when the long-pulsed PDL is used. They also agreed that "(1) acneiform flares may occur after any treatment, including ALA PDT, and (2) although not supported by extensive documentation, PDL activation provides the best results in ALA PDT for acne."

Randomized controlled studies of the use of MAL PDT for the treatment of acne vulgaris have been reported.[48,49] Horfelt and colleagues[48] found a statistically significant reduction in total inflammatory lesion count of patients treated with MAL PDT compared with placebo. Wiegell and Wulf[49] compared ALA and MAL in 15 patients with inflammatory acne and found that response rates were similar with both photosensitizing agents and that adverse effects were more prolonged and severe after ALA PDT. These conclusions were called into question by Gold,[50] who noted that Wiegell and Wulf's use of compounded ALA and the 3-hour incubation under occlusion were conditions not currently used in the United States for the treatment of acne by ALA PDT. Gold added that a more valid comparison would have used a commercially available ALA product (Levulan) incubated for 30 to 60 minutes without occlusion. Wiegell and colleagues[51] later reported that in tape-stripped normal skin, pain during and after illumination was greater with ALA PDT than with MAL PDT. Again, these investigators based their conclusions on the use of compounded ALA and the 3-hour incubation under occlusion.

In their evidence-based review of optical devices for the treatment of acne vulgaris, Haedersdal and colleagues[41] concluded that optical treatments offered short-term efficacy and that outcomes were the most consistent with PDT. They added that optically induced side effects, including pain, erythema, crusting, edema, hyperpigmentation, and pustular eruption, were more intense in PDT with ALA and MAL than with optical devices alone.

ACNE SCARS

Scarring occurs in 95% of patients with acne and in both sexes equally. The degree of scarring is related to the time delay in seeking treatment.[52] The decision on whether to treat a scar depends on the location of the scar, symptoms (itching, pain), severity of functional impairment (eg, joint mobility), and how distressed the patient is about the scar.[53] The modality used to treat the scar depends on the type of scar.[54] A simple system that classifies acne scars into icepick, rolling, or boxcar scars[55] is useful because it permits the clinician to distinguish between each type of scar by physical examination alone.

The 3 scar types differ in their width, depth, and three-dimensional architecture. Icepick scars occur at depths that exceed those reached by conventional resurfacing procedures, so they are best treated by punch excision. Boxcar scars can be treated by punch elevation; deep boxcar scars may also be treated by punch excision, and shallow boxcar scars respond well to laser resurfacing. Rolling scars are treated by subcision with or without laser resurfacing. Combinations of these 3 surgical procedures may also be necessary, followed by laser resurfacing some months later. Optimal results depend on accurate identification of the scar type[55] and response to a given treatment depends on the depth, degree of sclerosis, and location of the scar.[56] Atrophic and mixed patterns of facial acne scars have shown improvement when treated with a nonablative 1320-nm neodymium-doped:yttrium aluminum garnet (Nd:YAG) laser.[57]

Dermabrasion has been used to remove superficial scars and reduce the depth of deeper scars, but does not improve icepick scars.[11] It may also change pigmentation in darker-skinned people and has a lengthy learning curve.[58] Dermabrasion has been replaced by laser procedures in some countries.[54] The pulsed-dye 585-nm erbium-doped:yttrium aluminum garnet (Er:YAG) and CO_2 lasers are effective against superficial scars of facial acne.[54] Superficial chemical peeling may benefit icepick and U-shaped scars and is accompanied by reduced hyperpigmentation, reduced skin pore sizes, and improved complexion. Compared with superficial peeling, intermediate and deep peeling are associated with an increased risk of pigmentation and scarring.[11] Autologous fat, collagen, hyaluronic acid derivatives, and other biomaterials provide temporary improvement[11,54,59] in some scars.

Acne scars are the result of damage in and around the pilosebaceous follicle during inflammation.[60] The cause may be increased formation of tissue (hypertrophic scars and keloids) or loss or damage of tissue (icepick, rolling, boxcar scars).[54] Loss of collagen is also associated with acne scar formation[57,61] and the associated skin textural changes may be permanent.[62] Hypertrophic scars may occasionally resolve without intervention, whereas keloids are more persistent. Both may be treated singly or with a combination of excision, abrasion, laser devices and medication, and other modalities.[63] PIH, a brown or black discoloration in the area of a previous acne or other inflammatory lesion, is a common acne scar variant, particularly in dark-skinned patients. If protected from sun exposure, PIH appears 3 to 4 weeks after treatment[62] and fades in 3 to 18 months.[64] First-line therapies for PIH include chemical peels, bleaching agents, or lasers. Hypopigmentation, although rare,[62] may also result from acne lesions.[63] Hypertrophic scars, keloids, and pigmentary alterations may require medical interventions such as retinoids, topical or injectable steroids, silicone dressing, or other types of topical or injectable agents.[63] Intralesional injection of corticosteroids is a first-line treatment of keloids and second-line therapy for hypertrophic scars.[54] Cryotherapy before intralesional steroid injection induces fibrous tissue edema, which often permits injection of larger volumes of corticosteroids.[54] Combinations of various modalities have been recommended to maximize treatment efficacy for acne scars.[54,56,64] Current treatment modalities, including laser procedures, have been reviewed in detail.[62–65]

ACNE GRADING SCALES

The assessment of acne has been an evolutionary process that began with the publication of a 4-level grading system based on estimates of the number and types of lesions, the predominant lesion, and the degree of involvement.[14,66] Later schemes are shown in **Table 1**.

The complexity of acne (different lesion types at multiple skin sites; inter- and intrapersonal variations in the size, density, and severity of inflammation in localizad anatomic areas; and variability in natural healing and responses to therapy) contributes to the difficulty in classifying acne.[83] Grading severity on a scale such as 1 to 4 is subjective and considered simplistic. Other limitations of grading systems are that they require the user to undergo special training and that they are better suited for investigating new treatments than for use in the office setting.[14,83,84]

Standardized photographs used in some schemes may not reflect disease activity.[85] They also do not distinguish between macular and raised lesions, may not reveal small comedones and inflammatory lesions, do not permit palpation to determine the depth of involvement, and minimize the presence of residual erythema, tanned skin, pigmentary alterations, excoriations, and redness from light exposure.[14,83] Fluorescence and polar photography require special equipment and a considerable investment in time.[14]

In the authors' opinion, there is a need for a grading scale that offers strategies to assess and to treat acne in the office setting. Guidance is essential because acne is constantly changing and varies in presentation. Hormonal fluctuations, puberty, menopause, and stress present additional complexity. At-home regimens can be slow, frustrating, inadequate, and confusing, creating low compliance and poor results. Single device treatments may be ineffective because they address static and limited aspects of acne. Increasing resistance to antibiotics and awareness of side effects also pose challenges to oral and topical prescriptions.

Existing scales do not adequately guide treatments, especially when devices are used. Counting acne lesions is logistically challenging and results vary among practitioners. Existing global assessment scales lack critical procedural recommendations and do not address the multiple aspects of acne.

The authors have developed and validated a scale (**Table 2**) that addresses the shortcomings of existing scales. The Shamban Acne Scale (1) considers global assessment the major determinant of treatment, (2) suggests that a multimodal approach addressing the multiple aspects and variation of acne has the greatest practical relevance; (3) offers a guide to treatment, especially in the device category; (4) provides critical procedural recommendations, and (5) uses a novel photopneumatic system that synergizes light treatments with transdermal delivery of therapeutic substances.

As shown in **Table 2**, the Shamban Scale classifies acne according to 3 aspects: acne severity (A), scarring (S), and pigmentation (P). The bottom row of the table presents an example. In this case, the patient's acne is classified as A1-S2-P0. This means that acne severity is mild (1), scarring is moderate (2), and pigmentation abnormality is absent (0). With this information, the clinician can

Table 1
Grading systems for the assessment of acne[a]

Reference	Description
Pillsbury et al[66]	Clinical identification of lesions; 4 severity grades; no lesion counts
James and Tisserand[67]	Clinical identification of lesions; 4 severity grades; no lesion counts
Witkowski and Simona[68]	Clinical identification of lesions; lesions counted on one side of face
Burton et al[69]	Severity graded on scale of 0 (no lesions) to 5 (widespread inflammatory lesions and numerous larges cysts or pustules
Frank[70]	Numerical grading of each type of lesion on face, neck, back (0–4 and 0–10); 4 grades of overall severity
Plewig and Kligman[71]	Comedonal acne: overall severity grades 1–4 based on number of comedones on one side of face; papulopustular acne: overall severity grades 1–4 based on number of inflammatory lesions on one side of face
Christiansen et al[72]	Counted each type of lesion and total lesions; used area with most lesions as "test area": based response to treatment on reduction (%) of lesions in test area; graded reduction (%) on 6-point scale
Michaelson et al[73]	Assigned severity index to each type of lesion (comedones 0.5, papules 1.0, pustules 2.0, infiltrates 3.0, cysts 4.0); counted each type of lesion; multiplied severity index by lesion count for each lesion type; sum of products represented overall severity
Cook et al[74]	Overall numerical grade based on 5-point reference scale and 5 reference photographs of patients
Burke and Cunliffe[75]	Introduced Leeds technique of grading lesions (0–10) of face, chest, back and comparing results with reference photographs; used lesion counts, distinguished active from less active lesions on both sides of face
Samuelson[76]	Graded acne against a set of 9 reference photographs; response to treatment based on comparison with 9-grade scale at each visit
Lucchina et al[77]	Assessed severity of comedonal acne by fluorescent photography; scale 0–4
Lucky et al[78]	Counted lesions, recorded counts on facial template
Doshi et al[79]	Global Acne Grading System based on 6 anatomic areas, each assigned a numerical value based on its size; lesion types assigned numerical value based on severity; score for each area is the product of the area factor and the factor of the most severe lesion; total score is sum of products in each anatomic area; total score 1–18 = mild acne, 19–30 = moderate; 31–38 = severe, >39 = very severe
Dreno et al[80]	Similar to Doshi et al[79]
Phillips et al[81]	Severity of inflammatory acne based on photographs obtained with polarized light
Rizova and Kligman[82]	Assessed acne with photographs obtained with parallel and cross-polarized light, video microscopy, and measurements of sebum production

[a] Based on summary presented by Witkowski and Parish.[14]

Table 2
The Shamban Acne Scale

Acne	Scarring	Pigmentation
0. None	0. None	0. None
1. Mild	1. Mild	1. Mild
2. Moderate	2. Moderate	2. Moderate
3. Severe	3. Severe	3. Severe
A1	S2	P0

develop an in-office and at-home treatment plan that addresses scarring and acne lesions. Topical prescription agents include benzoyl peroxide, retinoids, dapsone, antibiotics, and azelaic acid, and oral agents include low-dose doxycyline, minocycline, oral contraceptives, spironolactone, and isotretinoin. As most acne treatments are effective in all skin types, skin color is not included in the new classification system.

To test the new system, the authors classified and treated 15 patients with varying degrees of inflammatory and papulopustular acne, old acne scars, and acne-induced pigmentation. Acne lesions were treated with light and acne therapeutic substances delivered transdermally, an oral prescription regimen, and a topical at-home regimen; old acne scars were treated with injectable fillers (hyaluronic acid, collagen, calcium hydroxyapatite, poly-L-lactic acid), punch elevation, punch excision, and a CO_2 laser device; and acne-induced pigmentation was treated with light and acne therapeutic substances delivered transdermally. Patients received 4 treatments at 2- to 3-week intervals.

Improvement of at least 1 grade in each aspect (acne, scarring, pigmentation) was observed in 90% of patients. At 1 month after the final treatment, 50% of patients improved 2 or more grades. Pore size reduction, skin texture improvement, and rhytid reduction were also observed. A clinical example is shown in **Fig. 1**.

Photopneumatic therapy combines the delivery of light with pneumatic energy. This novel modality has been introduced[86] and validated for the treatment of acne vulgaris.[50,87,88] The approach has been cleared by the FDA for the broadest acne indication –mild to moderate inflammatory acne (including acne vulgaris), comedonal acne, and pustular acne –as well as for the treatment of vascular and pigmented lesions. When the treatment tip makes complete contact with the skin, the vacuum is activated. The skin is gently stretched momentarily, increasing translucence by reducing the concentrations of hemoglobin and melanin. Light is then applied to the target tissue. The vacuum also exerts a mechanical pressure on the sebaceous gland, extruding the follicular ostia and evacuating sebaceous blockages. The result is more efficient photon delivery as a result of reduced absorption, reflection, and scatter by competing chromophores (melanin, hemoglobin). Stretching the skin reduces the concentration of melanin and blood cells, so the user can treat the target area with lower wavelengths of light for greater efficacy and with lower fluences for greater patient comfort during treatment. The Aesthera Isolaz™ system (Aesthera Corporation, Pleasanton, California) uses broadband light (400–1200 nm), which includes blue light for bacterial destruction and red light for its anti-inflammatory effects.[18,87] As indicated earlier, the vacuum of the Isolaz system evacuates the stebaceous gland. This is supported by an ultrastructural study[88] showing extrusion of comedo contents from the infundibulum of a sebaceous gland immediately after a single treatment and, 1 week after a second treatment, heat-induced injury to bacteria and necrosis of stratified epithelial cells in the lumina of pilosebaceous ducts.

The second part of the pneumatic device used in the present study is the profusion tip, which, while the skin is stretched, (topically) delivers proprietary therapeutic materials to the dermis via intercellular spaces and inverted pores. The combination of the Photpneumatic and PROFUSION Skin Therapy systems is the Isolaz Pro system (Aesthera Corporation). Treatment with the combined system requires 15 minutes without anesthesia or numbing creams.

To summarize, the device used in the present study stretches the skin, thereby lifting the sebaceous gland to the skin surface, cleanses the sebaceous gland, irradiates the cleansed gland with broadband light energy, and infuses the proprietary therapeutic substances into the cleansed gland.

The preliminary results of the present study show that the Shamban Acne Scale holds great

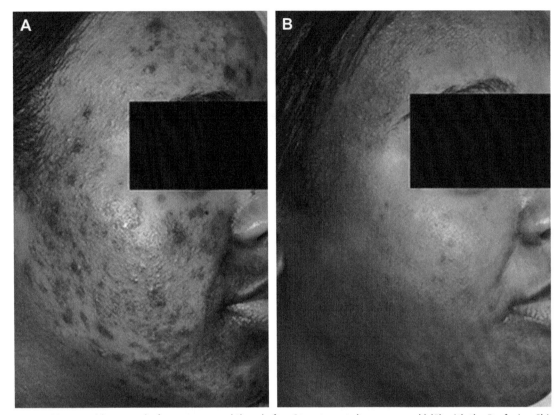

Fig. 1. A 23-year-old woman before treatment (*A*) and after 6 treatments (two per week) (*B*) with the Profusing Skin Therapy system (Aesthera Corporation, Pleasanton, CA). The patient's pretreatment classification using the Shamban Scale was A-2 (moderate acne), S-1 (mild scarring), P-3 (severe pigmentation). Pigmentation was treated by depigmentation (Cosmelan Peel). The patient's daily skin care regimen consisted of facial cleanser (NeosStrata), metranitazole gel (Metrogel, 1%, Galderma Laboratories, Fort Worth, TX), pimecrolimus (Elidel, Novartis Pharmaceuticals, East Hanover, NJ), and oil-free sunblock of SPF 45 (EltaMD) in the morning and facial cleanser, a gel mixture of clindamycin phosphate and tretinoin (Ziana, Medicis Dermatologics, Scottsdale, AZ), pimecrolimus, and a skin barrier emulsion (Epiceram, Promius Pharma, Bridgewater, NY) in the evening.

promise through improved use of multiple treatment modalities, simplification and combination of topical at-home therapies, design of complementary procedures for optimal results, and paves the way for biologic therapies.

SUMMARY

The Shamban Acne Scale is a useful guide in assessing and treating acne, acne-induced scars, and acne-induced pigmentation of varying severity in the office setting.

REFERENCES

1. Kraning KK, Odland GF. Prevalence, morbidity, and cost of dermatological diseases. J Invest Dermatol 1979;73(Suppl):395–401.
2. Leyden JJ. New understandings of the pathogenesis of acne. J Am Acad Dermatol 1995;32(5 Pt 3): S15–25.
3. Cunliffe WJ, Gould DJ. Prevalence of facial acne vulgaris in late adolescence and in adults. Br Med J 1979;1(6171):1109–10.
4. Gollnick H. Current concepts of the pathogenesis of acne: implications for drug treatment. Drugs 2003; 63(15):1579–96.
5. White GM. Recent findings in the epidemiologic evidence, classification, and subtypes of acne vulgaris. J Am Acad Dermatol 1998;39(2 Pt 3):S34–7.
6. Gollnick H, Cunliffe W, Berson D, et al. Global alliance to improve outcomes in acne. Management of acne: a report from a Global Alliance to Improve Outcomes in Acne. J Am Acad Dermatol 2003; 49(1 Suppl):S1–37.
7. Zaenglein AL, Thiboutot DM. Expert committee recommendations for acne management. Pediatrics 2006;118(3):1188–99.
8. Thiboutot DM. Overview of acne and its treatment. Cutis 2008;81(1 Suppl):3–7.
9. Guy R, Kealey T. Modelling the infundibulum in acne. Dermatology 1998;196(1):32–7.

10. Kim J. Review of the innate immune response in acne vulgaris: activation of Toll-like receptor 2 in acne triggers inflammatory cytokine responses. Dermatology 2005;211(3):193–8.

11. Dréno B, Bettoli V, Ochsendorf F, et al. European Expert Group on Oral Antibiotics in Acne. European recommendations on the use of oral antibiotics for acne. Eur J Dermatol 2004;14(6):391–9.

12. Strauss JS, Krowchuk DP, Leyden JJ, et al. American Academy of Dermatology/American Academy of Dermatology Association. Guidelines of care for acne vulgaris management. J Am Acad Dermatol 2007;56(4):651–63.

13. Shaw JC. Acne: effect of hormones on pathogenesis and management. Am J Clin Dermatol 2002;3(8):571–8.

14. Witkowski JA, Parish LC. The assessment of acne: an evaluation of grading and lesion counting in the measurement of acne. Clin Dermatol 2004;22(5):394–7.

15. Mills OH Jr, Kligman AM. Treatment of acne vulgaris with topically applied erythromycin and tretinoin. Acta Derm Venereol 1978;58(6):555–7.

16. Taub AF. Procedural treatments for acne vulgaris. Dermatol Surg 2007;33(9):1005–26.

17. Bhardwaj SS, Rohrer TE, Arndt K. Lasers and light therapy for acne vulgaris. Semin Cutan Med Surg 2005;24(2):107–12.

18. Papageorgiou P, Katsambas A, Chu A. Phototherapy with blue (415 nm) and red (660 nm) light in the treatment of acne vulgaris. Br J Dermatol 2000;142:973–8.

19. Kawada A, Aragane Y, Kameyama H, et al. Acne phototherapy with a high-intensity, enhanced, narrowband, blue light source: an open study and in vitro investigation. J Dermatol Sci 2002;30:129–35.

20. Elman M, Slatkine M, Harth Y. The effective treatment of acne vulgaris by a high-intensity, narrow band 405–420 nm light source. J Cosmet Laser Ther 2003;5:111–7.

21. Omi T, Bjerring P, Sato S, et al. 420 nm intense continuous light therapy for acne. J Cosmet Laser Ther 2004;6:156–62.

22. Tzung TY, Wu KH, Huang ML. Blue light phototherapy in the treatment of acne. Photodermatol Photoimmunol Photomed 2004;20:266–9.

23. Elman M, Lask G. The role of pulsed light and heat energy (LHE) in acne clearance. J Cosmet Laser Ther 2004;6:91–5.

24. Morton CA, Scholefield RD, Whitehurst C, et al. An open study to determine the efficacy of blue light in the treatment of mild to moderate acne. J Dermatolog Treat 2005;16:219–23.

25. Tremblay J, Sire D, Lowe N, et al. Light-emitting diode 415 nm in the treatment of inflammatory acne: an open-label, multicentric, pilot investigation. J Cosmet Laser Ther 2006;8:31–3.

26. Goldberg DJ, Russell BA. Combination blue (415 nm) and red (633 nm) LED phototherapy in the treatment of mild to severe acne vulgaris. J Cosmet Laser Ther 2006;8:71–5.

27. Gold M, Rao J, Goldman M, et al. Multicenter clinical evaluation of the treatment of mild to moderate inflammatory acne vulgaris of the face with visible blue light in comparison to topical 1% clindamycin antibiotic solution. J Drugs Dermatol 2005;4:64–70.

28. Sami NA, Attia AT, Badawi AM. Phototherapy in the treatment of acne vulgaris. J Drugs Dermatol 2008;7(7):627–32.

29. Patton T, Kress D. Light therapy in the treatment of acne vulgaris. J Cosmet Dermatol 2004;17(6):373–8.

30. González S, White WM, Rajadhyaksha M, et al. Confocal imaging of sebaceous gland hyperplasia in vivo to assess efficacy and mechanism of pulsed dye laser treatment. Lasers Surg Med 1999;25(1):8–12.

31. Seaton E, Charakida A, Mouser P, et al. Pulsed-dye laser treatment for inflammatory acne vulgaris: randomized controlled trial. Lancet 2003;362:1347–52.

32. Orringer J, Kang S, Hamilton T, et al. Treatment of acne vulgaris with a pulsed dye laser: a randomized controlled trial. JAMA 2004;291:2834–9.

33. Paithankar D, Ross E, Saleh B, et al. Acne treatment with a 1,450 nm wavelength laser and cryogen spray cooling. Lasers Surg Med 2002;31:106–14.

34. Friedman P, Jih M, Kimyai-Asadi A, et al. Treatment of inflammatory facial acne vulgaris with the 1450-nm diode laser: a pilot study. Dermatol Surg 2004;30:147–51.

35. Jih MH, Friedman PM, Goldberg LH, et al. The 1450-nm diode laser for facial inflammatory acne vulgaris: dose-response and 12-month follow-up study. J Am Acad Dermatol 2006;55:80–7.

36. Wang S, Counters J, Flor M, et al. Treatment of inflammatory facial acne with the 1,450 nm diode laser alone versus microdermabrasion plus the 1,450 nm laser: a randomized, split-face trial. Dermatol Surg 2006;32:249–55 [discussion: 255].

37. Lee CMW. Aura 532 nm laser for acne vulgaris—a three-year experience. Annual Combined Meeting of the American Society for Dermatologic Surgery and the American Society for Mohs Micrographic Surgery and Cutaneous Oncology, New Orleans, (LA), Oct 2003.

38. Baugh W, Kucaba W. Nonablative phototherapy for acne vulgaris using the KTP 532 nm laser. Dermatol Surg 2005;31:1290–6.

39. Glaich A, Friedman P, Jih M, et al. Treatment of inflammatory facial acne vulgaris with combination 595-nm pulsed-dye laser with dynamic-coolingdevice and 1,450-nm diode laser. Lasers Surg Med 2006;38:177–80.

40. Taylor MN, Gonzalez ML. The practicalities of photo-dynamic therapy in acne vulgaris. Br J Dermatol 2009;160:1140–8.

41. Haedersdal M, Togsverd-Bo K, Wulf HC. Evidence-based review of lasers, light sources and photody-namic therapy in the treatment of acne vulgaris. J Eur Acad Dermatol Venereol 2008;22(3):267–78.

42. Nestor M, Gold M, Kauvar A, et al. The use of photody-namic therapy in dermatology: results of a consensus conference. J Drugs Dermatol 2006;5:140–54.

43. Nestor MS. The use of photodynamic therapy for treatment of acne vulgaris. Dermatol Clin 2007; 25(1):47–57.

44. Kennedy J, Pottier R, Pross D. Photodynamic therapy with endogenous protoporphyrin IX: basic principles and present clinical experience. J Photo-chem Photobiol B 1990;6:143–8.

45. Divaris D, Kennedy J, Pottier R. Phototoxic damage to sebaceous glands and hair follicles of mice after systemic administration of 5-aminolevulinic acid correlates with localized protoporphyrin IX fluores-cence. Am J Pathol 1990;136:891–7.

46. Hongcharu W, Taylor C, Chang Y, et al. Topical ALA-photodynamic therapy for the treatment of acne vul-garis. J Invest Dermatol 2000;115:183–92.

47. Alexiades-Armenakas M. Long-pulsed dye laserme-diated photodynamic therapy combined with topical therapy for mild to severe comedonal, inflammatory, or cystic acne. J Drugs Dermatol 2006;5:45–55.

48. Hörfelt C, Funk J, Frohm-Nilsson M, et al. Topical methyl aminolaevulinate photodynamic therapy for treatment of facial acne vulgaris: results of a random-ized, controlled study. Br J Dermatol 2006;155(3): 608–13.

49. Wiegell SR, Wulf HC. Photodynamic therapy of acne vulgaris using 5-aminolevulinic acid versus methyl aminolevulinate. J Am Acad Dermatol 2006;54(4): 647–51.

50. Gold MH. 5-Aminolevulinic acid photodynamic therapy versus methyl aminolevulinate photody-namic therapy for inflammatory acne vulgaris. J Am Acad Dermatol 2008;58(2 Suppl):S60–2.

51. Wiegell SR, Stender IM, Na R, et al. Pain associated with photodynamic therapy using 5-aminolevulinic acid or 5-aminolevulinic acid methylester on tapes-tripped normal skin. Arch Dermatol 2003;139(9): 1173–7.

52. Layton AM, Henderson CA, Cunliffe WJ. A clinical evaluation of acne scarring and its incidence. Clin Exp Dermatol 1994;19(4):303–8.

53. Bayat A, McGrother DA, Ferguson MWJ. Skin scar-ring. BMJ 2003;326:88–92.

54. Jemec GB, Jemec B. Acne: treatment of scars. Clin Dermatol 2004;22:434–8.

55. Jacob CE, Dover JS, Kaminer MS. Acne scarring: a classification system and review of treatment options. J Am Acad Dermatol 2001;45:109–17.

56. Hirsch RJ, Lewis AB. Treatment of acne scarring. Semin Cutan Med Surg 2001;20:190–8.

57. Rogachefsky AS, Hussain M, Goldberg DJ. Atrophic and mixed pattern of acne scars improved with a 1320-nm Nd:YAG laser. Dermatol Surg 2003;29: 904–8.

58. Swinehart JM. Case reports: surgical therapy of acne scars in pigmented skin. J Drugs Dermatol 2007;6:74–7.

59. Lee DH, Choi YS, Min SU, et al. Comparison of a 585-nm pulsed dye laser and a 1064-nm Nd:YAG laser for the treatment of acne scars: A randomized split-face clinical study. J Am Acad Dermatol 2009; 60:801–7.

60. Holland DB, Jeremy AH, Roberts SG, et al. Inflam-mation in acne scarring: a comparison of the responses in lesions from patients prone and not prone to scar. Br J Dermatol 2004;150:72–81.

61. Cunliffe WJ, Simpson NB. Disorders of the sebaceoud glands. In: Champion RH, Burton JL, Burns DA, editors. Rook/Wilkinson/Ebling textbook of derma-tology. Oxford: Blackwell Science; 1998. p. 1927–84.

62. Alster T, Zaulyanov L. Laser scar revision: a review. Dermatol Surg 2007;33:131–40.

63. Rivera AE. Acne scarring: a review and current treat-ment modalities. J Am Acad Dermatol 2008;59: 659–76.

64. Goodman GJ. Postacne scarring: a review of its pathophysiology and treatment. Dermatol Surg 2000;26:857–71.

65. Tanzi EL, Alster TS. Laser treatment of scars. Skin Therapy Lett 2004;9:4–7.

66. Pillsbury DM, Shelley WB, Kligman AM. Derma-tology. Philadelphia: Saunders; 1956. p. 810.

67. James K, Tisserand JJ. Treatment of acne vulgaris. GP 1958;18:131–9.

68. Witkowski JA, Simons HM. Objective evaluation of demethylchlortetracycline hydrochloride in the treat-ment of acne. JAMA 1966;196:397–400.

69. Burton JI, Cunliffe WJ, Stafford I, et al. The preva-lence of acne vulgaris in adolescence. Br J Dermatol 1971;85:119–26.

70. Frank SB. Acne vulgaris. Springfield (IL): Thomas; 1971. p. 12–3.

71. Plewig G, Kligman A. Acne: morphogenesis and treatment. New York: Springer-Verlag; 1975. p. 162–3.

72. Christiansen J, Holm P, Reymann F. Treatment of acne vulgaris with retinoic acid derivative Ro 11-1430. A controlled clinical trial against retinoic acid. Dermatologica 1976;153:172–6.

73. Michaelson G, Juhlin L, Bahlquist A. Oral zinc sulphate therapy for acne vulgaris. Acta Derm Vene-reol 1977;57:372.

74. Cook CH, Centner RL, Michaels SE. An acne grading method using photographic standards. Arch Dermatol 1979;115:571–5.

75. Burke BM, Cunliffe WJ. The assessment of acne vulgaris: the Leeds technique. Br J Dermatol 1984;111:83–92.

76. Samuelson JS. An accurate photographic method for grading acne: initial use in a double-blind clinical comparison of minocycline and tetracycline. J Am Acad Dermatol 1985;12:461–7.

77. Lucchina LC, Kollias N, Phillips SB. Quantitative evaluation of noninflammatory acne with fluorescence photography. J Invest Dermatol 1994;102:560.

78. Lucky AW, Barber BL, Girman CJ, et al. A multirater validation study to assess the reliability of acne lesion counting. J Am Acad Dermatol 1996;35:559–65.

79. Doshi A, Zaheer A, Stiller MJ. A comparison of current acne grading systems and proposal of a novel system. Int J Dermatol 1997;36:416–8.

80. Dreno B, Godokh I, Chivot M, et al. ECLA grading: a system of acne classification for everyday dermatological practice. Ann Dermatol Venereol 1999;126:136–41.

81. Phillips SB, Kollias N, Gillies R, et al. Polarized light photography enhances visualization of inflammatory lesions of acne vulgaris. J Am Acad Dermatol 1997;37:948–52.

82. Rizova E, Kligman A. New photographic techniques for clinical evaluation of acne. J Eur Acad Dermatol Venereol 2001;15(Suppl 3):13–8.

83. Pochi PE, Shalita AR, Strauss JS, et al. Report of the Consensus Conference on Acne Classification. Washington, D.C., March 24 and 25, 1990. J Am Acad Dermatol 1991;24:495–500.

84. Shalita AR, Leyden JJ Jr, Kligman AM. Reliabilty of acne lesion counting. J Am Acad Dermatol 1997;37:672.

85. Pochi PE. The pathogenesis and treatment of acne. Annu Rev Med 1990;41:187–98.

86. Narurkar VA. Novel photopneumatic therapy delivers high-efficiency photos to dermal targets. J Cosmet Dermatol 2005;18(2):115–20.

87. Shamban AT, Enokibori M, Narurkar V, et al. Photopneumatic technology for the treatment of acne vulgaris. J Drugs Dermatol 2008;7(2):139–45.

88. Omi T, Munavalli GS, Kawana S, et al. Ultrastructural evidence for thermal injury to pilosebaceous units during the treatment of acne using photopneumatic (PPX) therapy. J Cosmet Laser Ther 2008;10:7–11.

Nonablative Fractional Laser Resurfacing

Vic A. Narurkar, MD[a,b,c,*]

KEYWORDS
- Farctional laser resurfacing • Nonablative lasers

Fractional photothermolysis is an extension of selective photothermolysis, which is the fundamental mechanism for most laser and light-based devices. Despite the safety of selective photothermolysis, there remained a risk of bulk heating, regardless of whether ablative and nonablative modes of laser delivery were employed. The development of nonablative fractional photothermolysis was motivated by two factors—a safer mode for skin resurfacing compared with traditional ablative laser resurfacing and a more effective mode for skin resurfacing, compared with largely ineffective nonablative methods of resurfacing. Several wavelengths have been used for nonablative fractional resurfacing (NFR), and some novel wavelengths are under clinical development for enhancing efficacy, while maintaining safety. Finally, combination therapies of NFR with nonablative skin tightening devices may act synergistically for global facial and nonfacial rejuvenation.

THE SCIENCE OF NONABLATIVE FRACTIONAL LASER RESURFACING

The fundamental concept behind all nonablative fractional laser devices involves three criteria including (1) the creation of microthermal zones of damage to the treated tissue, (2) extrusion of contents with a true resurfacing, and (3) rapid reepithelialization within 24 hours. Manstein and colleagues[1] first reported the concept of fractional photothermolysis for cutaneous applications using an array of microscopic thermal zones (MTZ) with a prototype 1550 nm erbium-doped laser. This approach was defined as NFR. NFR creates small

volumes of thermal damage within the skin, allowing for rapid epidermal repair because of smaller epidermal wounds and a rapid migratory path for keratinocytes. In contrast to purely nonablative resurfacing, which was generally clinically unimpressive, NFR created essential epidermal extrusion for resurfacing effects, while confining dermal thermal damage. The latter, which was primarily the mechanism of pure nonablative resurfacing, produced impressive histologic findings but limited clinical findings. Macroablative laser resurfacing, which produced both impressive clinical and histologic findings, had significant risks including hypopigmentation, persistent erythema, and hypertrophic scarring. NFR creates microscopic patterns of laser wounds that produce spheroid segments of epidermal necrotic debris with relative preservation of the stratum corneum.[2] Dermal effects of microthermal zone repair generate wound mediators that ultimately lead to remodeling of the dermal matrix and histologic demonstration of enhanced rete ridge patterning and increased mucin production, which augment skin rejuvenation. The most widely studied device for NFR employs a 1550 nm erbium-doped laser with a random scanning pattern. Other devices that use NFR include a 1540 nm laser with a stamped pattern of microthermal injury, a 1410 nm laser using a random scanning pattern of injury, and a 1440 nm laser with a stamped pattern of microthermal injury (**Table 1**).

CLINICAL INDICATIONS FOR NFR

NFR has expanded the use of clinical indications compared with traditional macroablative laser

[a] Department of Dermatology, California Pacific Medical Center, San Francisco, CA, USA
[b] Bay Area Laser Institute, San Francisco, CA, USA
[c] Department of Dermatology, University of California Davis School of Medicine, Sacramento, CA, USA
* Department of Dermatology, University of California Davis School of Medicine, Sacramento, CA.
E-mail address: vicnarurkar@yahoo.com

Dermatol Clin 27 (2009) 473–478
doi:10.1016/j.det.2009.08.012
0733-8635/09/$ – see front matter © 2009 Published by Elsevier Inc.

derm.theclinics.com

Table 1
Other devices that use NFR

NFR Device	Mechanism	Example
1410 nm	Random scanning to create microthermal zones	Fraxel refine
1440 nm	Stamped pattern to create microthermal zones	Cynosure affirm
1540 nm	Stamped pattern to create microthermal zones	Palomar Starlux 1540
1550 nm	Random scanning to create microthermal zones	Fraxel restore

resurfacing and enhanced the efficacy of clinical indications compared with traditional nonablative laser resurfacing.[3,4] **Table 2** summarizes the clinical indications for NFR with levels of efficacy and safety. The first indications of NFR were the treatment of periorbital rhytids and benign pigmented lesions. Since its inception, the clinical indications have expanded tremendously. The optimal clinical indications for NFR include photoaging; dyshchromias; acne scarring (distensible, nondistensible, and ice pick); surgical and traumatic scars such as burn scars; and mild to moderate Glogau photoaging of the face, neck, chest and other body locations. NFR is also effective for therapy-resistant melasma, moderate to severe photoaging of facial and nonfacial skin, and striae distensae. The least efficacy of NFR has been shown to be moderate to severe perioral rhytids and significant laxity. For these indications, traditional macroablative laser resurfacing and fractional ablative laser resurfacing may be better alternatives.

NFR treatment of dyschromias is based on the creation of microscopic epidermal necrotic debris that also contains melanin pigment. The proposed mechanism is a type of so-called melanin shuttle that is extruded. Along with the dermal remodeling effects and extrusion of dermal content such as elastin fibers, the global effect of NFR is the gradual reversal of the combined increased epidermal pigmentation and solar elastosis of photoaging. Moreover, this approach can be used on both facial and nonfacial skin because the predominant mechanism is nonablative, thereby reducing bulk heating, which is the limiting factor of off face laser treatments. Three to five treatments, spaced over 4 to 6 weeks, produce impressive results for dyschromia using NFR devices (**Fig. 1**).

Acne scarring treatments have been generally disappointing using traditional laser therapy, with the exception of traditional macroablative lasers, which pose significant risks. Moreover, most treatments require subcision and excision of certain types of scars in addition to resurfacing, and are generally unimpressive for ice pick acne scars. NFR devices are effective for multidimensional acne scarring, including distensible acne scars, nondistensible acne scars, ice pick scars, and scars with erythema and postinflammatory hyperpigmentation. Acne scars typically require more treatments than treatment of photodamage. All skin types can be treated effectively if appropriate parameters are used (**Fig. 2**), with reduction of treatment densities to avoid pigmentary issues.

Surgical and traumatic scars such as burn scars have shown impressive results with NFR.[5] The unique aspect of NFR compared with other devices is the ability to treat hypopigmented scars. Before the development of NFR, treatment of

Table 2
Clinical indications for NFR

Indication	Efficacy
Acne scars	++++
Surgical and traumatic scars	++++
Dyschromia or photodamage face	+++
Dyschromia orphotodamage off face	+++
Melasma	++
Striae distensae	++
Deep rhytids and laxity	+

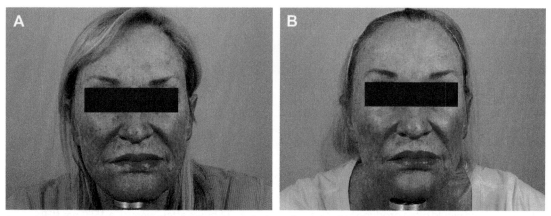

Fig. 1. (*A*) Before 1550 nm NFR for dyschromia and photodamage. (*B*) After 1550 nm NFR for dyschromia and photodamage.

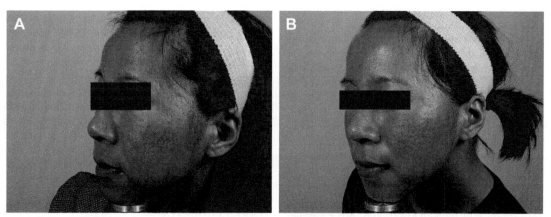

Fig. 2. (*A*) Acne scars before 1550 nm NFR; skin type V. (*B*) Acne scars after three 1550 nm NFR treatments; skin type V.

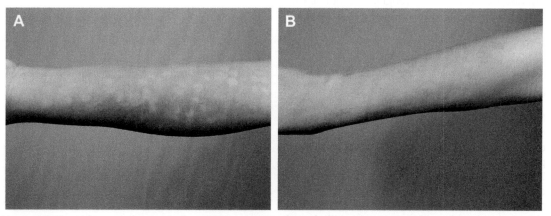

Fig. 3. (*A*) Hypopigmented scars before 1550 nm NFR. (*B*) Hypopigmented scars after three 1550 nm NFR treatments.

hypopigmented scars was generally disappointing. NFR devices can improve young and mature hypopigmented scars (**Fig. 3**). The mechanism for improvement may involve recruitment of melanin from surrounding skin through the melanin shuttle.

Nonfacial resurfacing with NFR is gaining momentum, as there are limited options for treatment of the neck, chest, hands, and beyond. Poikiloderma of Civatte is a typical condition of the neck, which is better treated with NFR because it represents a multifocal problem: erythema and dyschromia due to both melanin and hemosiderin.[6] Before NFR, the mainstay of treatment of poikiloderma of Civatte was limited to pulsed dye lasers and intense pulsed light, and would often produce honeycombing or rectangular patterns. NFR has increased both the safety and efficacy of the treatment of poikiloderma of Civatte. In addition to the improvement of the dyschromia of the neck, NFR also improves the global texture through collagen remodeling. A similar mechanism is useful for NFR treatment of the aging chest and hands.

The treatment of melasma is one of the greatest challenges in dermatology. Melasma is notorious for recurrence and resistance. Laser therapy of melasma has traditionally been disappointing and can actually exacerbate melasma. Of all devices, NFR-based devices offer the greatest hope for treating therapy-resistant melasma.[7] The approach should be conservative, and the use of lower fluencies and treatment densities are warranted. The patient also needs to be informed of the recurrence of melasma. Aggressive before and after skin care, including sunscreens and bleaching creams, are essential for successful outcomes.

Moderate to deep perioral rhytides and laxity is not very successful with NFR devices, although some degree of improvement can be seen. If NFR is to be used for moderate to deep perioral rhytides, it is best done in conjunction with dermal fillers and botulinum toxin. NFR will produce modest improvement in laxity; however, if NFR is to be used for laxity, it is best done in conjunction with skin-tightening devices.

PATIENT SELECTION AND PREPARATION FOR NFR

NFR has expanded the use of lasers in all Fitzpatrick skin types.[1–4,6–9] There have been no reports of hypopigmentation or depigmentation. Transient postinflammatory hyperpigmentation can be seen, but prevented, using lower fluencies and treatment densities and preparing the skin with bleaching creams and sunscreen. All patients, regardless of skin type, should wear sunscreens with broad spectrum UV-A and UV-B coverage before

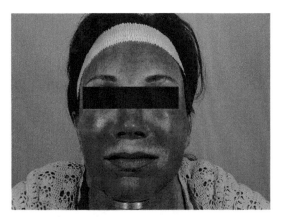

Fig. 4. 72-hours after aggressive 1550 nm NFR.

treatment, during the course of treatments, and after treatments. Darker skin types should all be pretreated with hydroquinones for at least 3 to 4 weeks before treatment. Test sites are always advisable as they can be used to optimize treatment parameters. Retinoids should be discontinued several days before treatment, as blistering has been reported in patients who were on topical retinoic acid creams during treatments. For facial treatments, oral herpes simplex virus (HSV) prophylaxis with valacyclovir of famciclovir is indicated, regardless of a history of oral HSV. If patients give a history of recurrent HSV, it is advisable to continue treatment with antivirals for 3 to 5 days after treatment, particularly for more aggressive resurfacing parameters.

POSTTREATMENT CARE FOR NFR

NFR devices will produce rapid reepithelialization. However, patients show varying degrees of recovery after treatment, particularly in regards to edema (**Fig. 4**). Therefore, it is important to

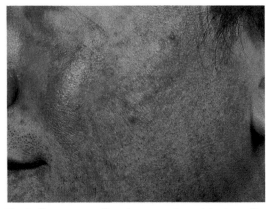

Fig. 5. Recurrence of melasma and persistent postinflammatory hyperpigmentation after 1550 nm NFR.

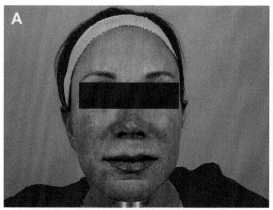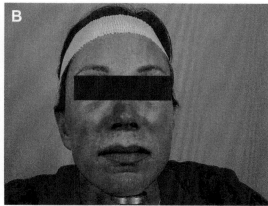

Fig. 6. (A) Before unipolar radiofrequency and 1550 nm NFR. (B) After unipolar radiofrequency and 1550 nm NFR.

discuss a posttreatment plan with patients. Some pre- and posttreatment skin care regimens have been studied with NFR, including a probiotic skin care line and Biafine cream, both showing enhanced recovery after treatment. One hundred percent of patients will experience posttreatment edema, in the range from 24 hours to 7 days. Posttreatment erythema is also very common, but usually resolves in 2 to 4 days. Acneiform eruptions—particularly in the perioral area—are common, with rates ranging from 10% to 20%, and are self-limiting. However, if a patient gives a history of acne vulgaris, it is reasonable to treat with oral antibiotics during the posttreatment phase. Xerosis and pruritus occur in 3 to 4 days and quickly resolve. The average time for NFR recovery is 2 to 4 days, compared with 7 to 21 days for macroablative laser resurfacing.

COMPLICATIONS

Complications with NFR devices are rare and generally self-limiting.[10] The majority of complications are technique or parameter related. Blistering has been reported, particularly if higher fluencies and treatment densities are used with excessive overlap of delivery. They generally heal without scarring. Prolonged erythema has been reported with higher fluencies, but generally resolves. Microthermal zone pattern persistence can occur (more with stamping devices), particularly off-face and resolves within 2 to 3 weeks. Petechiae and pinpoint hemorrhaging can be seen in thinner skin areas such as eyelid and periorbital skin, and in striae. Scarring is exceedingly rare and usually a result of overaggressive treatments and overlapping pulses. Postinflammatory hyperpigmentation and melasma recurrence can be seen (Fig. 5) and generally managed with the tincture of time

and bleaching creams. Hypopigmentation and depigmentation with NFR has not been reported.

FUTURE DIRECTIONS

To address limitations of NFR, several strategies have been developed, including the use of synergistic devices for improvement of laxity and the introduction of newer wavelengths for enhancing efficacy. The former has been studied with the combined 1440 nm fractional laser and a 1320 nm laser, and combining a 1550 nm fractional laser with unipolar radiofrequency (Fig. 6).[11] These approaches employ NFR devices to address surface anomalies and a complimentary device (1320 nm laser; unipolar radiofrequency) to address laxity. Recently, a 1927 nm thulium nonablative, fractionated laser has been developed to address recurrence of dyschromia, resistant melasma, and the need for fewer treatments. This modality can be considered an intermediary device between NFR and ablative fractional resurfacing (AFR). While AFR may be less risky than traditional macroablative resurfacing, it still is ablative and carries greater downtime and risks. The intermediary approach may enhance the efficacy of NFR, but retain the safety.

SUMMARY

NFR uses a nonablative mode of delivery with preservation of the stratum corneum, a true resurfacing with epidermal extrusion, and creation of microscopic thermal zones of injury that ultimately lead to neocollagenesis. The most impressive clinical results are seen with acne scars, surgical and traumatic scars, and mild to moderate facial and nonfacial dyschromia or photoaging. Modest results can be seen with therapy-resistant melasma and certain types of rhytides. Future approaches include synergistic treatments with radiofrequency devices and the development of novel wavelengths to enhance the efficacy of NFR while preserving safety.

REFERENCES

1. Manstein D, Herron GS, Sink RK, et al. Fractional photothermolysis: a new concept for cutaneous remodeling using microscopic patterns of thermal injury. Lasers Surg Med 2004;34:426–38.
2. Laubach H, Tannous Z, Anderson R, et al. Skin responses to fractional photothermolysis. Lasers Surg Med 2006;38(2):142–9.
3. Wanner M, Tanzi E, Alster T. Fractional photothermolysis: treatment of facial and nonfacial cutaneous photodamage with a 1550 nm erbium-doped fiber laser. Dermatol Surg 2007;33:23–8.
4. Laubach HJ, Tannous Z, Anderson RR, et al. A histological analysis of the dermal effects after fractional photothermolysis treatment. Lasers Surg Med 2005;36(S17):86.
5. Glaich AS, Rahman Z, Goldberg LH, et al. Fractional resurfacing for the treatment of hypopigmented scars: a pilot study. Dermatol Surg 2007;33:298–301.
6. Behroozan D, Goldberg LH, Glaich AS, et al. Fractional photothermolysis for the treatment of poikiloderma of Civatte. Dermatol Surg 2006;32:298–301.
7. Rokhsar C, Fitzpatrick R. The treatment of melasma with fractional photothermolysis: a pilot study. Dermatol Surg 2005;31:1645–50.
8. Narurkar VA. Skin rejuvenation with microthermal fractional photothermolysis. Dermatol Ther 2007;20:S10–3.
9. Geronemus RG. Fractional photothermolysis: current and future applications. Lasers Surg Med 2006;38:169–76.
10. Graber EM, Tanzi EL, Alster TA. Side effects and complications of fractional photothermolysis. Experience with 961 treatments. Dermatol Surg 2008;34:301–7.
11. Geraghty LN, Biesman B. Clinical evaluation of a single wavelength fractional laser and a novel multiwavelength fractional laser in the treatment of photodamaged skin. Lasers Surg Med 2009;41(6):408–16.

Ablative and Fractional Ablative Lasers

Lori A. Brightman, MD[a,b,]*, Jeremy A. Brauer, MD[c],
Robert Anolik, MD[c], Elliot Weiss, MD[a], Julie Karen, MD[a,c],
Anne Chapas, MD[a,c], Elizabeth Hale, MD[a,c],
Leonard Bernstein, MD[a], Roy G. Geronemus, MD[a,c]

KEYWORDS
- Laser rejuvenation • Ablative laser
- Fractional ablative laser • Resurfacing • Nonablative

As we age, skin texture and tone responsible for youthful elasticity and complexion deteriorate. Photodamage augments these changes, while other insults, such as scars from surgery, trauma, and acne, further burden skin appearance. Consequently, demand is strong for safe and effective treatments to bolster underlying tissue and mitigate these unwanted visible changes. Laser resurfacing has proven to be a powerful technique for achieving these goals. Through innovations, laser resurfacing has established an improved safety profile and attracted greater attention.

Laser resurfacing for rejuvenation was first widely offered in the 1980s using ablative carbon dioxide (CO_2) lasers. The technology is based on the theory of selective photothermolysis. Briefly, this involves the delivery of a specific wavelength of light absorbed by select molecules, or chromophores.[1,2] Delivering wavelengths of 10,600 nm, these CO_2 lasers specifically targeted water as their chromophore. The lasers wiped away the entire epidermis, along with some of the dermis, which allowed for improved tone and texture upon reepithelialization.

For years, the fully ablative CO_2 laser was the gold standard in skin resurfacing. However, the side effect profile demanded the development of alternative approaches, despite various enhancements and their proven effectiveness in the treatment of rhytides, photodamage, and scars.[3–5] Nonablative laser resurfacing systems were introduced, but yielded comparatively mild clinical improvement. In 2004, the concept of fractional photothermolysis was introduced. In photothermolysis, only a specific fraction of the epidermal and dermal architecture is treated.[6] The untouched intervening areas allow for a more rapid repopulation of the epidermis and a less significant side effect profile when compared with confluent ablative resurfacing. Moreover, fractional resurfacing offers significantly better outcomes than those seen with nonablative methods. Its ample clinical improvement, when combined with its relatively safe side effect profile, has propelled fractional ablative laser resurfacing into the forefront of skin rejuvenation.

ABLATIVE LASERS
History

CO_2 laser resurfacing, introduced in the 1980s, is built on the foundation of selective photothermolysis.[1,2] Modifications to the CO_2 laser, as well as the introduction of erbium-doped yttrium aluminum garnet (Er:YAG) lasers, provide clinicians with a number of options when choosing to treat patients with ablative technologies.

Technology

Delivering 10,600-nm wavelengths in the far-infrared electromagnetic spectrum, CO_2 lasers target water. Consequently, they penetrate

[a] Laser & Skin Surgery Center of New York, 317 East 34th Street, New York, NY 10016, USA
[b] Department of Plastic Surgery and Reconstructive Surgery, New York Eye and Ear Infirmary, Dermatology Services, 310 East 14th Street, New York, NY 10003, USA
[c] The Ronald O. Perelman Department of Dermatology, New York University School of Medicine, 560 First Avenue # H-100, New York, NY 10016, USA
* Corresponding author. Laser & Skin Surgery Center of New York, 317 East 34th Street, New York, NY 10016.
E-mail address: lbrightman@laserskinsurgery.com (L.A. Brightman).

Dermatol Clin 27 (2009) 479–489
doi:10.1016/j.det.2009.08.009
0733-8635/09/$ – see front matter © 2009 Elsevier Inc. All rights reserved.

without regard to melanin and hemoglobin. At fluences of 5 J/cm^2, the vaporization threshold of tissue, and pulse durations of less than 1 ms, the thermal relaxation time of tissue, optical penetration is 20 to 30 μm.[7–9] Residual thermal damage extends to about 100 to 150 μm.[7–9] When CO_2 lasers fail to deliver a fluence that surpasses the vaporization threshold, they instead coagulate and desiccate the tissue.[10] Fluence is directly affected by the beam diameter. Initial commercially available devices included some small-diameter beams (100–300 μm) that achieved high fluences with rapid vaporization, while larger (2 mm) diameter beams often led to relatively more thermal heating and subsequent charring, especially when not rapidly moved over the target field.

The necessary ablation parameters were first achieved using two separate CO_2 strategies. One was a high-power, individually pulsed CO_2 laser that could deliver 500 mJ in 600 μs to 1 ms. When administered in a 3-mm spot or in a specific computer pattern generator made up of dozens of 2.25-mm spots, sufficient fluences greater than 5 J/cm^2 were achieved.[11] The other strategy for attaining the ablation parameters involved a lower-energy, rapidly scanning continuous-wave CO_2 laser. This method focused small-diameter beams to generate sufficient fluence and scanned them in several nonoverlapping shapes. At dwell times less than a millisecond, fluence rose above ablation threshold.

Further developments in ablative technology led to the Er:YAG laser, emitting wavelengths at 2940 nm. Although sharing water as a target chromophore, Er:YAG lasers demonstrate more precise ablation when compared with the CO_2 laser. This results from its closer approximation to the absorption peak of water of 3000 nm, resulting in a more limited depth of penetration and essentially no thermal damage. Laser penetration is only 1 to 3 μm per J/cm^2, with residual thermal damage only reaching 10 to 40 μm.

In general, the CO_2 laser and the Er:YAG laser offer similar cosmetic results, but comparative studies tend to favor the former.[12,13] Subsequent modifications of the Er:YAG lasers have offered additional treatment options to the dermatologic surgeon, including the development of a variable-pulse Er:YAG. This technology enables the surgeon to vary pulse duration from one that is primarily ablative to one that is more thermal, resulting in fewer side effects than those related to CO_2 treatments.[12]

Plasma skin resurfacing is a relatively new non-ablative and fully ablative strategy. This technology is based on delivery of high-energy radiofrequency into nitrogen gas, which generates nitrogen plasma targeted at the treatment area.[14] Heat is transferred to the skin, driving the collagen denaturation and subsequent neocollagenesis. Early studies show improvement in photodamage and scars, even on nonfacial surfaces.[14,15] In a plasma skin resurfacing study of 10 patients, 30 areas with evidence of photodamage, including sites on the neck, chest, and dorsal hand, were randomly selected for treatment with one of three energy settings.[14] Digital photographs and independent clinical evaluations before, immediately after, and at posttreatment days 4, 7, 14, 30, and 90 demonstrated a statistically significant reduction in wrinkle severity ($P<.001$) and hyperpigmentation ($P<.001$), as well as increased skin smoothness ($P<.05$). Additionally, punch biopsies obtained from each of the 30 areas 90 days after treatment revealed epidermal thickening, decreased solar elastosis, and increased amount of new collagen deposition. Although promising, this technology has not yet been fully evaluated in comparison to the CO_2 and Er:YAG lasers.

Histology

The histology of skin treated with laser ablation has been well studied and varies based on study and device used. Some lasers ablate the entire epidermis with one pass, while others may leave areas of dermoepidermal junction intact, requiring further passes, depending upon desired depth of treatment.[7]

The histologic effects of ablative laser therapy were assessed in a study of 33 patients randomized to receive treatment of forehead, glabella, periorbital, or perioral regions with either or both the high-power, individually pulsed CO_2 laser and a lower-energy, rapidly scanning continuous-wave CO_2 laser.[16] Biopsies were performed on the skin of seven individuals before, immediately after, and 1 year after a minimum of three passes.

The sizes of the subepidermal repair zone and the zone of dermal fibrosis deep to the dermoepidermal junction were measured in all specimens. Preoperative specimens demonstrated degrees of solar elastosis that correlated with the level of clinical photodamage. Those specimens with evidence of the most severe photodamage showed focal effacement of the rete ridges, as well as vacuolated keratinocytes in the epidermis. A pretreatment Grenz zone of varying thickness (10–40 μm) was noted between this zone of solar elastosis and the epidermis.

Immediately after treatment, specimens were evaluated for collagen thermal damage, with the use of polarization birefringence for verification of depth. Thermal damage extended from 70 to 180 μm into the dermis, with preservation of at least the base of the dermal papillae in most cases, suggesting that no more than 80 μm of the dermis was ablated. Biopsy specimens obtained after 1 year showed a zone of horizontally arranged collagen fibers measuring 100 to 350 μm. The thickness of the layer of solar elastosis was decreased compared with the thickness seen in preablation specimens.

Indications

Ablative laser resurfacing enables physicians to aggressively treat a number of concerns. A primary indication is photoaging, which includes rhytides, dyspigmentation, vascular changes, elastosis, actinic cheilitis, and actinic keratoses. Another common indication for ablative resurfacing is scarring, such as that incurred from acne, surgery, and trauma.

Both photoaging and scars respond well to ablative resurfacing, but the degree of scar response notably varies with type.[3–5] A retrospective study of 47 patients with perioral, periorbital, and glabellar rhytides demonstrated good to excellent cosmetic results in all anatomic areas after treatment with a CO_2 laser with a scanning device.[3] Similar findings were reported in a study of photodamaged perioral and periorbital skin treated with a pulsed CO_2 laser.[4] Clinical evaluation revealed the removal of superficial wrinkles, and a significant improvement in deeper ones. Additionally a tightening of previously loose and folded skin was observed.

Fifty patients with moderate to severe atrophic facial acne scars enrolled in a study involving high-energy, pulsed CO_2 laser.[5] Independent and blind clinical and photographic assessments were made in all patients. Furthermore, textural analysis of pretreated and treated skin was performed on a smaller subset of the subjects, for confirmation of clinical impressions. The observers ultimately reported greater than an eighty percent average clinical improvement in acne scars.

Ice-pick scars from severe acne tend not to respond as well, but the incorporation of other strategies, such as subcision and punch excisions before laser resurfacing deliver improved outcomes.[17] Traumatic and surgical scars have been shown to respond well to ablative resurfacing, particularly when treated 6 to 10 weeks after the insult.

In the setting of a dermatologic surgery practice, ablative resurfacing may be considered following perceptible Mohs micrographic surgery scars,

debulking of hypertrophic scars, and thickened graphs, for example. Other indications include exophytic lesions, such as rhinophyma, warts, and adnexal tumors, as well as bothersome benign hamartomas, such as epidermal nevi.[18]

In a case series of 10 patients—5 with inflammatory linear verrucous epidermal nevus and 5 with linear verrucous epidermal nevus—subjects underwent CO_2 laser treatment at 20 W and with a 200-mm hand piece.[18] A minimum of two passes and maximum of eight, over four sessions, were applied to each area. Despite such side effects as scarring and hyperpigmentation, several patients achieved complete removal without recurrence by the end of their observation period.

Patient Selection

Careful consideration is imperative when determining which patient is a candidate for ablative laser resurfacing. Patient expectation, skin type and medical history should be thoroughly assessed before initiation.

An ideal patient has reasonable expectations for cosmetic outcome. Patients should understand the side effect profile, as discussed later, as well as be able to manage the necessary downtime following treatment. The patient should understand that, because of greater risks of scarring, some areas will not be treated. Those areas include the neck, chest, and hands. The ideal patient is of Fitzpatrick skin type I through IV, and has a primary concern cited or related to the indications described above.

Because certain histories can directly, and negatively, influence outcome, a patient's medical history plays a critical role in patient selection. A patient with history of keloids should not undergo the procedure, as the procedure may trigger another keloidal response. Similarly, patients with dermatologic diseases that demonstrate koebnerization, such as vitiligo, lichen planus, and psoriasis, should be cautioned and likely dissuaded from undergoing ablation.

Any suggestion of adnexal disease also serves as a contraindication to ablative laser resurfacing. Ablative resurfacing relies on the repopulation of the epidermis from stem cells found in skin appendages. A deficiency of these appendages, as seen in morphea and scleroderma, for example, serve as contraindications because of their diminished stem cell supply. Furthermore, while the number of sebaceous glands remains approximately the same throughout life, they tend to increase in size with age, and therefore younger patients may not be as suited to this form of treatment.

Several iatrogenic conditions can also serve as contraindications. Skin treated with radiation therapy should not undergo ablation for the same rationale just cited: namely, a relative absence of adnexal structures to repopulate the epidermis. Recent treatment with isotretinoin also serves as a contraindication, since atypical scarring has been reported in dermabrasion and chemical peeling following its use.[19] Though not evidence-based, many consider a wash-out period of at least 1 year as adequate when treating patients who have been on isotretinoin.[20] Finally, ablative resurfacing after extensive surgical procedures is also contraindicated. It is not uncommon for patients seeking ablative laser resurfacing to have had surgical face-lifts and blepharoplasties. In fact, they may seek this treatment immediately after or even during these invasive procedures. However, the altered blood supply, as a result of surgical undermining and skin repositioning, puts the skin at greater risk for necrosis and scarring.[20]

Perioperative Management and Anesthesia

Oral antiviral and antibacterial prophylaxis is generally recommended to prevent herpes and secondary bacterial eruptions.[21] Commonly, anti-herpetic agents, such as acyclovir or valacyclovir, are administered 1 day before treatment and continued until reepithelialization is complete, usually under 2 weeks. Prophylactic antibiotics of choice are usually penicillins or macrolides. For prevention of secondary candida or other fungal infections, some prescribe antifungals, such as flu-conazole, although these are much less commonly employed.[22] Ironically, despite the contraindication to ablative laser resurfacing following systemic retinoid treatment, preoperative topical retinoids, often tretinoin, are often recommended. Tretinoin is thought to prime the skin for more rapid healing after ablation.[23]

To counter the chance for significant edema, some practitioners prescribe systemic corticosteroids prophylactically, which extend over a few days following treatment.

Options for anesthesia exist over a wide spectrum, from topical agents and local infiltration to nerve blocks and systemic agents. Patient tolerance, treatment area, and technology employed all influence the decision. The CO_2 laser is thought to be more painful than the Er: YAG laser because of the greater tissue-heating effect on type C pain fibers. Superficial laser procedures, particularly short-pulsed Er:YAG treatments, are often managed with topical agents, such as lidocaine and prilocaine cream. These can be combined with local infiltration of anesthetic, particularly

when treating a specific cosmetic unit. When broadly treating the central forehead, median cheek, nose, upper lip, lower lip, and/or chin, a variety of blocks, including supraorbital, supratro-chlear, infraorbital, and mental nerve blocks may be employed as appropriate. Blocks may be achieved simply using lidocaine 1% to 2% with 1:100,000 or 1:200,000 epinephrine, but can be enhanced by bu-pivicaine 0.5%, 1:10 sodium bicarbonate ($NaHCO_3$) 8.4% to neutralize the pH and, subsequently, diminish pain. Patients undergoing total face resurfacing and patients who are particularly sensitive may warrant the addition of systemic agents as well, including anxiolytics, narcotics, intramuscular sedation, or intravenous anesthesia.

Postoperative management includes the acute care of edema, exudate, and skin sloughing. If the edema is severe enough, oral corticosteroids may be prescribed over a short term. Cool compresses, head elevation, soaks in saline or water, and protection with a petrolatum ointment as well as biooclusive dressings are additionally methods of caring for these patients postoperatively. In light of the incidence of allergic contact dermatitis to these agents and the prophylactic oral antibiotics most patients are already using, petrolatum ointment is generally preferred over topical antibiotics.

Erythema of the treated areas can possibly persist for months, so patients should be advised to use makeup with green tints. Additionally, patients must be strongly advised to use sunscreen and practice sun protective behavior to reduce risks of postinflammatory hyperpigmentation.

Complications

The relatively high incidence of side effects and lengthy recovery period following treatment has transitioned ablative laser resurfacing into a less favorable light. Still, it has a role in dermatologic surgery. Therefore, a thorough appreciation for its side effect profile is warranted. The most notable and well-documented complications of laser ablation resurfacing are scarring and delayed-onset hypopigmentation, although a more exhaustive discussion of complications follows here.

Scarring after laser ablation is the result of excessive ablation and thermal damage. Although aggressive treatments with high-energy fluences, excessive treatment passes, and the overlap of treatment passes—so-called "pulse stacking"—produce more dramatic outcomes, these actions also amplify the potential risk of scar. Therefore, the expertise of the practitioner, to carefully balance the risks and benefits of these parameters, is paramount. Proper postoperative wound care also plays a role in scar formation.

Delayed-onset hypopigmentation is another conspicuous concern. Two forms of hypopigmentation are described following laser ablative resurfacing. Relative hypopigmentation consists of hypopigmentation in relation to background, untreated skin.[24] These complications are often managed and less noticeable by treating cosmetic units or the entire face and feathering treatment into surrounding areas. Delayed-onset hypopigmentation, on the other hand, develops 6 to 12 months after initial treatment. These permanent changes have been described in up to 57% of patients.[25] In addition to creating a new cosmetic concern, the change draws attention to areas of the body that are already unacceptable to the patient, areas in which the patient just underwent treatment.

Hyperpigmentation may also develop, particularly in darker skin types. This tends to favor more superficial ablation, while deeper passes favor hypopigmentation.

Other recognized complications of ablative laser resurfacing are generally self-limited and resolve with appropriate care. Erythema, resulting from laser-induced inflammation, is part of the normal healing process. Resolution occurs over a few months but can last up to a year. These changes may be exacerbated with exertion or emotional volatility, though they can be masked by green-tinted makeup.

Acneiform eruptions are thought to stem from follicular reepithelialization and the occlusive ointments and dressings related to wound management.[3] Fortunately, these normally respond to standard acne treatments, although isotretinoin is avoided because of its association with atypical scarring in resurfacing procedures.

An eczematous dermatitis may develop, which is generally responsive to topical corticosteroids.[3] Furthermore, some have reported an incidence of perioral dermatitis following treatment, which responds well to oral doxycycline.

Finally, superficial herpetic and bacterial eruptions can result, though the use of prophylactic antivirals and antibiotics have resulted in fewer reported episodes.[21] Rarely, fungal eruptions, such as candidiasis, may present, which can be treated with standard courses of fluconazole.[22]

NONABLATIVE LASERS

Demand for a better side effect profile and minimal downtime fueled the rapid advent of newer technologies, as well as superior modifications and adaptations of older ones. In particular, nonablative lasers were developed, along with fractionated variants of ablative lasers. While a lengthy discussion of nonablative lasers is beyond the scope of this review, they deserve mention.

The method of damage is perhaps the major difference between these technologies. Nonablative lasers heat but do not ablate. The mode of delivery of the heat can be in a stamping or rolling application for ablative and nonablative lasers.[26] Ablative and fractional ablative lasers result in epidermal vaporization and dermal coagulation in all affected areas. This is in stark contrast to nonablative devices with complete protection of the epidermis secondary to laser type, settings, and cooling mechanisms.[26]

The greatest advantage to nonablative lasers over their ablative and fractional ablative counterparts is their more attractive side effect profile. However, efficacy of a single treatment may be considered less than ideal. It is the responsibility of the physician to be certain the patient has reasonable expectations and may require a series of treatments to achieve desired outcome.

FRACTIONAL ABLATIVE LASERS
History

Until recently, ablative laser resurfacing served as the primary method to achieve moderate or greater resurfacing outcomes. In the last several years, however, the theory of fractional photothermolysis, pioneered by Anderson and colleagues,[27] along with the technology of traditional ablative lasers, has spawned the rise of the field of fractional ablative therapy.

Technology

Fractional technologies deliver columns of spatially confined thermal injury to the skin, in what are known as microthermal zones, thereby avoiding confluent epidermal damage. The surrounding unaffected follicular units and their stem cells, as well as available fibroblasts, aid in rapid repopulation and collagen remodeling of these zones. The first lasers employing this concept were the nonablative fractional technologies, such as the 1550-nm erbium-doped fiber laser, which yielded relatively minimal downtime and mild erythema. However, as previously described, the results obtained with nonablative resurfacing, including those with fractional technology, were still inferior to ablative strategies. The natural progression of technology along with the continued desire for superior results led to the combination of the theory of fractional photothermolysis and ablative laser technologies.

Nearly 20 independent laser suppliers, and over twice as many actual products and hand pieces have been created to take advantage of the new fractional technology. The major differences among devices pertain to the depth of ablation and coagulation and the variations in treatment hand pieces, with their varying spot sizes and shapes, as well as mode of application (rolling or stamping). Treatment hand pieces vary according to the manner in which the treatments are performed and delivered to microthermal zones. Examples, of such hand pieces include those shaped to apply fractional ablative lasers for treating eyeliner or lipliner cosmetic tattoos (**Fig. 1**). Device types include fractional 532-nm diode, 850- to 1350-nm infrared, 1064-nm/2940-nm Er:YAG, 1550-nm erbium-fiber, 2790-nm yttrium scandium gallium garnet (YSGG), 10,600-nm CO_2, and radiofrequency lasers and hand pieces. These products emit different pulse lengths and different amounts of energy.

Histology

Histologic studies examining fractional ablative devices have demonstrated that typical microthermal zones consist of a tapered ablative zone, surrounded by eschar and a thermal coagulation zone, with maximum lesion depths ranging from 300 μm to over 1 mm and lesion widths of 140 μm to almost 300 μm.[6,28] More recently, it has been reported that fractional ablative lasers can achieve a depth of over 1.5 mm into the dermis at higher energy levels (70 mJ).[29] Furthermore, re-epithelialization was shown to be complete in a matter of 2 days, with extrusion of the coagulated tissue, or microepidermal necrotic debris.[28,30] This debris forms beneath the intact corneal layer above each dermal wound, marking the transition of keratinocyte function to wound repair. As these necrotic elements contain melanin, a mild bronze color developed and persisted up to weeks after treatment. Lastly, enhancement of the superficial dermal rete and deposition of mucin were also identified.

Indications

Fractional ablative technologies have been successfully used in the treatment of a variety of scars, including acne,[30,31] surgical, and traumatic scars[32]; in the treatment of facial rhytides and photodamaged skin[33]; and for debulking. Furthermore, anecdotal evidence suggests efficacy with actinic cheilitis, residua of infantile hemangiomas, cosmetic treatment of lower-eyelid bags, and repigmentation of areas of delayed-type hypopigmentation that followed fully ablative laser resurfacing treatments.[29] Perhaps these observed repigmentation effects are secondary to a decreased definition or demarcation of the hypopigmented area or, more remarkably, a renewed stimulation of melanocytes.

Ablative fractional resurfacing has been demonstrated to both normalize the skin topography of both atrophic and hypertrophic scars.[29] In a study of 15 subjects with Fitzpatrick skin types I through IV and moderate to severe acne scarring, all patients experienced an average of 66.8% improvement in depth of their acne scars after two to three full-face treatments with a fractional CO_2 laser.[31] Additionally, these individuals experienced a 26% to

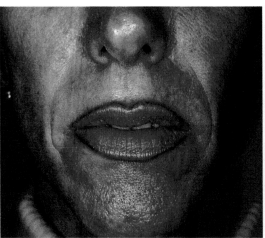 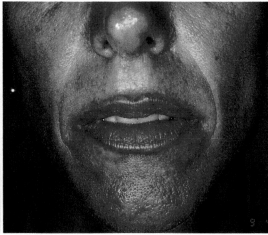

Fig. 1. Vermillion border cosmetic tattoo removal with fractional CO_2 laser. (*Data from* Mafong E, Kauvar ANB, Geronemus RG. Surgical pearl: Removal of cosmetic lip-liner tattoo with the pulsed carbon dioxide laser. Journal of the American Academy of Dermatology 2003;48(2):271–2.)

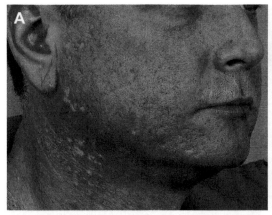 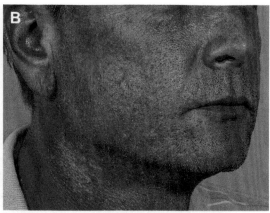

Fig. 2. Acne scarring reduction with fractional CO_2 laser. (A) Baseline. (B) Three months postprocedure.

50% improvement in texture, atrophy, and overall improvement of scarring when evaluated by both investigators as well as themselves (Fig. 2).

In a recent letter to the editor, one investigator reported a case of a man with a 5-year-old thermal burn wound on the upper extremity with skin grafting that left an uneven texture and "mesh"-like pattern that was successfully treated with fractional CO_2 laser.[32] Three side-by-side test areas were created, one with medium-density microthermal zones, one with high-density microthermal zones, and a control. Assessment was made 3 months after treatment, and a significant improvement in texture and color of the skin treated with the high-density coverage was seen, with skin texture, in particular, appearing distinctly more even and smooth compared with that of the control area. Additionally, a slight improvement was noted in the area treated with the medium-density coverage. Although each case must be

independently evaluated for treatment, the recommendation for scars is for a series of two to four treatments with 6 to 12 weeks between treatments.

Fine and moderate facial rhytides as well as many signs of photodamage, including solar elastosis, laxity, and lentigines, have been successfully treated with fractional ablative resurfacing. A series of 32 patients, each treated with a microablative CO_2 laser, was reported. The investigators evaluated the effects on wrinkles, acne scars, striae, lentigines, and solar elastosis.[33] These subjects, with Fitzpatrick skin types I through III, underwent a single laser resurfacing treatment of either the face, neck, trunk, or extremities. Photographs taken at 1, 2, 3, 12, and 24 weeks, as well as patient-satisfaction survey responses, were analyzed. According to the investigators, the best results were seen in wrinkles, lentigines, and solar elastosis, with less-impressive effects on striae and acne scarring (Figs. 3–7).

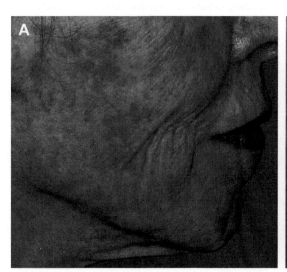 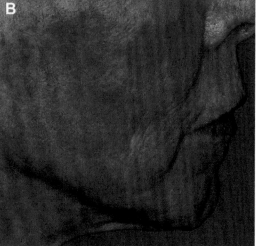

Fig. 3. Subject treated with fractional CO_2 laser. (A) Baseline. (B) One-month follow-up postprocedure.

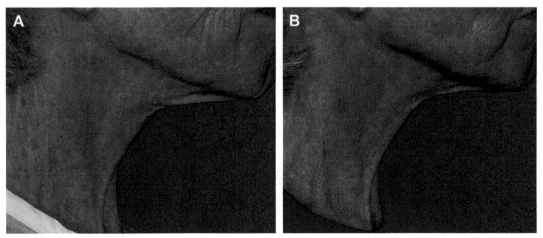

Fig. 4. Subject treated with fractional CO_2 laser. (*A*) Baseline. (*B*) Neck rejuvenation and subsequent submentum tightening.

As mentioned, scarring secondary to surgery has been successfully treated with fractional ablative lasers. In many cases, these scars are the result of several surgeries, including debulking procedures. Laser surgery may prevail in this arena, not only because of promising results, but because the emotional toll of numerous scalpel-based surgeries may yield patients more amenable to lasers than other interventions (**Fig. 8**).

Patient Selection

Proper patient selection is vital to the success of any resurfacing procedure. A patient considering fractional ablative laser resurfacing should be evaluated in the same way a patient would be who was considering fully ablative laser resurfacing. Notably, however, fractional laser treatments offer far greater flexibility in patients of all skin types and ages, as well as in those desiring treatment of

body areas other than the face. In-office protocols may certainly vary. However, the protocols described below are fairly common.

Perioperative Management and Anesthesia

As discussed, for management of individuals undergoing ablative procedures, prophylaxis, both antibiotic and antiviral, must be considered, depending upon the patient's history. It is generally accepted that all patients, with or without a past medical history of herpes labialis, begin antiviral therapy, as well as prophylactic antibiotics, 1 day prior through 5 days after therapy. A several-day course, usually a week or slightly more, should also be initiated 1 day before the procedure.

During fractional ablative resurfacing, cold-air cooling is used to maximize comfort. Topical anesthetic agents, such as lidocaine and prilocaine creams, are often applied 60 minutes before the

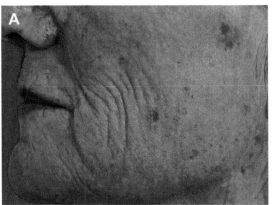
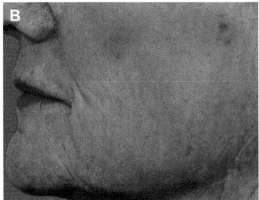

Fig. 5. Subject treated with fractional CO_2 laser. (*A*) Baseline. (*B*) Three-month follow-up postprocedure.

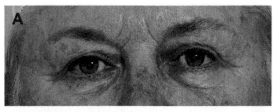 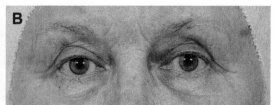

Fig. 6. Subject treated with fractional CO_2 laser for periorbital rejuvenation with noted reduction of upper-eyelid hooding, rhytids, infraorbital tear-trough discoloration, and crepelike skin. (*A*) Baseline. (*B*) Three-month postprocedure.

procedure. Nerve blocks, in particular surpaorbital, infraorbital, and mental nerve blocks, are administered 15 minutes before the procedure.[29] Less commonly, some physicians prefer to perform full-face treatments with intravenous sedation and in the presence of an anesthesiologist.

Technique, of course, is highly variable and is physician- and device-parameter–dependent. Sequential treatment of cosmetic units—the cheeks, nose, lips, chin, temples, forehead, and eyelids—is performed with each pass perpendicular to the last to minimize bulk heating. These treatments result in immediate edema, oozing, pinpoint bleeding, and crusting at higher settings.

Postoperatively, ice-cold soaks may be applied, followed by application of a petrolatum ointment. The patient is bandaged with a protective sterile mask, escorted home, and instructed to keep the face moist at all times until crusting has resolved, which on average is by day 3, at which point they may begin a nongreasy moisturizing cream. Reports have also advocated administration of

oral prednisone 30 mg the morning of the procedure, as well as the following 2 days, if the patient continues to experience significant edema or the procedure involved the upper cheeks and lower eyelids.[29,30] Sun avoidance and protection is important in minimizing postinflammatory hyperpigmentation.

Complications

The chief advantage of fractional ablative resurfacing when compared with fully ablative alternatives is its side effect profile matched with its proven, ample effectiveness. Most notable is its lower risk of scarring on both facial and nonfacial skin and its lower risk of hypopigmentation, particularly permanent, delayed-type hypopigmentation. Safe and effective treatments may involve the neck, chest, back, and extremities.[30,33] Fully ablative treatments on nonfacial areas, on the other hand, can lead to scarring and hyperpigmentation, with the possibility of permanence and disfigurement.

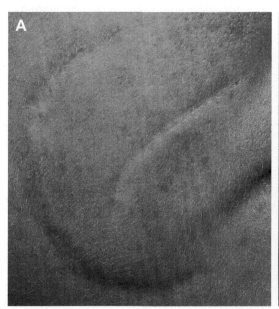 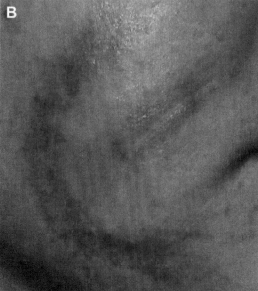

Fig. 7. Significant improvement in left buccal cheek scar that occurred 18 years before treatment. (*A*) Baseline. (*B*) One-month post–second treatment with fractional CO_2 laser.

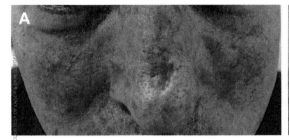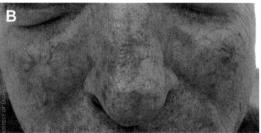

Fig. 8. Atrophic Mohs micrographic scar improved with fractional CO_2 laser treatment. (A) Baseline. (B) Three months posttreatment.

This is likely due to lower hair-follicle density, and therefore availability of stem cells, as well as a less-extensive vascular supply. In our office, with well over 1000 patients treated, there has not been a reported case of scarring or hypopigmentation to date. In fact, only a few cases of fractional ablative resurfacing–related scarring have been reported in the literature, and these cases are likely secondary to improper technique or overuse of energy and density settings. Three of four cases in one report involved scarring after treatment of the neck for skin laxity and melasma.[34,35] The fourth was a case of ectropion and lower-eyelid scarring after treatment for facial rhytides.[34,35]

SUMMARY

The field of nonsurgical laser resurfacing for aesthetic enhancement continues to improve with new research and technological advances. Since its beginnings in the 1980s, the laser-resurfacing industry has produced a multitude of devices employing ablative, nonablative, and fractional ablative technologies. The three approaches differ largely in their method of thermal damage, weighing degrees of efficacy, downtime, and side effect profiles against each other. Nonablative technologies generate some interest, although only for those patient populations seeking mild improvements. Fractional technologies, however, have gained dramatic ground on fully ablative resurfacing. Despite exhibiting results that fall just short of the ideal outcomes of fully ablative treatments, fractional laser resurfacing is an increasingly attractive alternative because of its far more favorable side effect profile, reduced recovery time, and significant clinical outcome.

REFERENCES

1. Altshuler GB, Anderson RR, Manstein D, et al. Extended theory of selective photothermolysis. Lasers Surg Med 2001;29:416–32.

2. Anderson RR, Parrish JA. Selective photothermolysis: precise microsurgery by selective absorption of pulsed radiation. Science 1983;220:524–7.

3. Waldorf HA, Kauvar AN, Geronemus RG. Skin resurfacing of fine to deep rhytides using a char-free carbon dioxide laser in 47 patients. Dermatol Surg 1995;21:940–6.

4. Fitzpatrick RE, Goldman MP, Satur NM, et al. Pulsed carbon dioxide laser resurfacing of photo-aged facial skin. Arch Dermatol 1996;132:395–402.

5. Alster TS, West TB. Resurfacing of atrophic facial acne scars with a high-energy, pulsed carbon dioxide laser. Dermatol Surg 1996;22:151–4.

6. Manstein D, Herron GS, Sink RK, et al. Fractional photothermolysis: a new concept for cutaneous remodeling using microscopic patterns of thermal injury. Lasers Surg Med 2004;34:426–38.

7. Kauvar AN, Waldorf HA, Geronemus RG. A histopathological comparison of "char-free" carbon dioxide lasers. Dermatol Surg 1996;22:343–8.

8. Green HA, Domankevitz Y, Nishioka NS. Pulsed carbon dioxide laser ablation of burned skin: in vitro and in vivo analysis. Lasers Surg Med 1990;10:476–84.

9. Walsh JT Jr, Flotte TJ, Anderson RR, et al. Pulsed CO2 laser tissue ablation: effect of tissue type and pulse duration on thermal damage. Lasers Surg Med 1988;8:108–18.

10. Kauvar AN, Geronemus RG. Histology of laser resurfacing. Dermatol Clin 1997;15:459–67.

11. Yang CC, Chai CY. Animal study of skin resurfacing using the ultrapulse carbon dioxide laser. Ann Plast Surg 1995;35:154–8.

12. Newman JB, Lord JL, Ash K, et al. Variable pulse erbium: YAG laser skin resurfacing of perioral rhytides and side-by-side comparison with carbon dioxide laser. Lasers Surg Med 2000;26:208–14.

13. Khatri KA, Ross V, Grevelink JM, et al. Comparison of erbium: YAG and carbon dioxide lasers in resurfacing of facial rhytides. Arch Dermatol 1999;135:391–7.

14. Alster TS, Konda S. Plasma skin resurfacing for regeneration of neck, chest, and hand: investigation of a novel device. Dermatol Surg 2007;33:1315–21.

15. Kono T, Groff WF, Sakurai H, et al. Treatment of traumatic scars using plasma skin regeneration (PSR) system. Lasers Surg Med 2009;41:128–30.

16. Ross EV, Grossman MC, Duke D, et al. Long-term results after CO2 laser skin resurfacing: a comparison of scanned and pulsed systems. J Am Acad Dermatol 1997;37:709–18.

17. Jacob CI, Dover JS, Kaminer MS. Acne scarring: a classification system and review of treatment options. J Am Acad Dermatol 2001;45:109–17.

18. Michel JL, Has C, Has V. Resurfacing CO2 laser treatment of linear verrucous epidermal nevus. Eur J Dermatol 2001;11:436–9.

19. Rubenstein R, Roenigk HH Jr, Stegman SJ, et al. Atypical keloids after dermabrasion of patients taking isotretinoin. J Am Acad Dermatol 1986;15:280–5.

20. Hayes DK, Berkland ME, Stambaugh KI. Dermal healing after local skin flaps and chemical peel. Arch Otolaryngol Head Neck Surg 1990;116:794–7.

21. Nestor MS. Prophylaxis for and treatment of uncomplicated skin and skin structure infections in laser and cosmetic surgery. J Drugs Dermatol 2005;4:s20–5.

22. Conn H, Nanda VS. Prophylactic fluconazole promotes reepithelialization in full-face carbon dioxide laser skin resurfacing. Lasers Surg Med 2000;26:201–7.

23. Alt TH. Technical aids for dermabrasion. J Dermatol Surg Oncol 1987;13:638–48.

24. Bernstein LJ, Kauvar AN, Grossman MC, et al. The short- and long-term side effects of carbon dioxide laser resurfacing. Dermatol Surg 1997;23:519–25.

25. Dijkema SJ, van der Lei B. Long-term results of upper lips treated for rhytides with carbon dioxide laser. Plast Reconstr Surg 2005;115:1731–5.

26. Hantash BM, Mahmood MB. Fractional photothermolysis: a novel aesthetic laser surgery modality. Dermatol Surg 2007;33:525–34.

27. Huzaira M, Anderson RR, Sink K, et al. Intradermal focusing of near-infrared optical pulses: a new approach for non-ablative laser therapy. Lasers Surg Med 2003;32(Suppl 15):17–38.

28. Hantash BM, Bedi VP, Kapadia B, et al. In vivo histological evaluation of a novel ablative fractional resurfacing device. Lasers Surg Med 2007;39(2):96–107.

29. Hunzeker CM, Weiss ET, Geronemus RG. Fractionated carbon dioxide laser resurfacing: our experience with more than 2,000 treatments. Aesth Surg Journal, in press.

30. Geronemus RG. Fractional photothermolysis: current and future applications. Lasers Surg Med 2006;38:169–76.

31. Chapas AM, Brithman L, Sukal S, et al. Successful treatment of acneiform scarring with CO2 ablative fractional resurfacing. Lasers Surg Med 2008;40:381–6.

32. Hædersdal M. Fractional ablative CO(2) laser resurfacing improves a thermal burn scar. J Eur Acad Dermatol Venereol 2009 [epublication].

33. Gotkin RH, Sarnoff DS, Cannarozzo G, et al. Ablative skin resurfacing with a novel microablative CO2 laser. J Drugs Dermatol 2009;8:138–44.

34. Fife DJ, Fitzpatrick RE, Zachary CB. Complications of fractional co2 laser resurfacing: four cases. Lasers Surg Med 2009;41:179–84.

35. Ross RB, Spencer J. Scarring and persistent erythema after fractional ablative CO2 laser resurfacing. J Drugs Dermatol 2008;7:1072–3.

Tissue Tightening Technologies

Melissa A. Bogle, MD[a,b,*], Jeffrey S. Dover, MD, FRCPC[c,d,e]

KEYWORDS

- Tissue tightening • Radiofrequency • Skin tightening
- Laxity • Rejuvenation

Surgical intervention is the gold standard for correction of skin laxity on the face and the body. While there is no comparison to the dramatic improvements that can be accomplished with surgical procedures, many patients see the recovery time, risk, and high expense as significant drawbacks to this approach. Patients and cosmetic physicians have become more savvy about skin rejuvenation and aging. Many patients would rather have less invasive, less expensive procedures done with less downtime and more natural looking results. They not only want to avoid the risks of surgery, such as permanent nerve injury, skin flap necrosis, and visible scars, but they also do not want to look like they have obviously had a procedure. While there is a trade off in the amount of skin tightening that can be achieved with nonsurgical techniques, there is a high market demand for the procedure. The key is in selecting suitable patients, setting appropriate expectations, and combining nonsurgical skin-tightening technologies with other modalities, such as fillers and botulinum toxin, to enhance the overall result.

RADIOFREQUENCY ENERGY: BACKGROUND SCIENCE

Nonsurgical approaches to skin tightening have been widely researched and now there are several approaches. The first modality marketed specifically for noninvasive skin tightening was radiofrequency energy. Radiofrequency energy is a form of electromagnetic energy ranging from 300 MHz to 3 kHz. The technology has been used in many areas of medicine including cardiology, urology, and sleep medicine. In dermatology the technology has been used for electrocoagulation, hemostasis, endovenous closure, and skin rejuvenation.[1]

Radiofrequency energy is similar to laser and light energy in that its interaction with tissue induces thermal changes, however it does not follow the principles of selective photothermolysis. Rather than inducing heat by selectively targeting a particular chromophore, radiofrequency devices generate heat as a result of tissue resistance to the movement of electrons within the radiofrequency field (Ohm's law) (**Fig. 1**).[1]

Essentially, radiofrequency devices work by using a generator to produce an alternating current that creates an electric field through the skin. The electric field shifts polarity millions of times per second, causing a change in the orientation of charged particles within the electric field. It is the tissue resistance to this particle movement that generates heat in the skin. Thus, heat is generated by the skin's resistance to the flow of current within an electric field, not by photon absorption as with a laser.[1] While certain lasers, such as those in the infrared spectrum, are able to affect upper

The authors have no funding support to disclose.

a The Laser and Cosmetic Surgery Center of Houston, 3700 Buffalo Speedway, Suite 700, Houston, TX 77098, USA
b Department of Dermatology, The University of Texas M.D. Anderson Cancer Center, 6655 Travis Street, Suite 980, Houston, TX 77030, USA
c Skin Care Physicians, 1244 Boylston Street, Chestnut Hill, MA 02467, USA
d Section of Dermatologic Surgery and Oncology, Department of Dermatology, Yale University School of Medicine, 333 Cedar Street, LCI 501, New Haven, CT 06520, USA
e Department of Dermatology, Dartmouth Medical School, One Medical Center Drive, Hanover, NH 03756, USA
* Corresponding author. The Laser and Cosmetic Surgery Center of Houston, 3700 Buffalo Speedway, Suite 700, Houston, TX 77098.

Dermatol Clin 27 (2009) 491–499
doi:10.1016/j.det.2009.08.008
0733-8635/09/$ – see front matter © 2009 Elsevier Inc. All rights reserved.

$$\text{Energy} = I^2 \times Z \times t$$

Fig. 1. Ohm's Law states the impedance (Z) to the movement of electrons creates heat relative to the amount of current (I) and time (t). Energy = $I^2 \times Z \times t$.

dermal collagen and improve fine wrinkles and textural irregularities, they are less suited to adequately address the problem of deep or subdermal skin laxity. Energy from laser or light sources tends to scatter or absorb in the upper layers of the skin, making it difficult to deliver sufficient energy to the deep dermis without causing damage.[1] While these differences caused early efforts at noninvasive skin tightening to focus mainly on radiofrequency devices, research has now expanded out to include other modalities able to penetrate into the deep layers of the skin and soft tissue such as ultrasound energy which will be discussed later in the article.

The depth of energy delivered by a radiofrequency device depends on several factors including the arrangement of radiofrequency electrodes (ie, either monopolar or bipolar), the type of tissue serving as the conduction medium (ie, fat, blood, skin), temperature, and the frequency of the electrical current applied.[1]

The arrangement of electrodes in a radiofrequency device can be either monopolar or bipolar (**Fig. 2**). The two systems create different electromagnetic fields, however the interaction of the energy with the target tissue is similar. In a monopolar system, the electrical current passes through a single electrode in the hand piece to a grounding pad. Without appropriate surface cooling, there is a high density of power close to the electrode's surface and a deep power penetration. If the operator is not careful, this can lead to safety concerns, such as burns or overheating and high pain levels.[1-3] In a bipolar system, the electrical current passes between two electrodes at a fixed distance over the skin. The advantage to this is that there is a more controlled current distribution. The main disadvantage is that the penetration depth of the energy into the tissue is limited to roughly half the distance between the electrodes.[1,2]

Electrical conductivity varies among different types of tissue and even from patient to patient and under different operating conditions. Not all patients will have the same amount of energy deposited in a particular area with otherwise equal parameters. The structure of each individual's tissue (dermal thickness, fat thickness, fibrous septa, number, and size of adnexal structures) all play a role in determining impedance and heat perception.[1,4,5] In general, blood has a very high electrical conductivity, while fat, bone and dry skin have lower conductivities so that the current tends to flow around the structures rather than passing through them. Wet skin has a higher electrical conductivity than dry skin, which is why improved results can be seen with generous

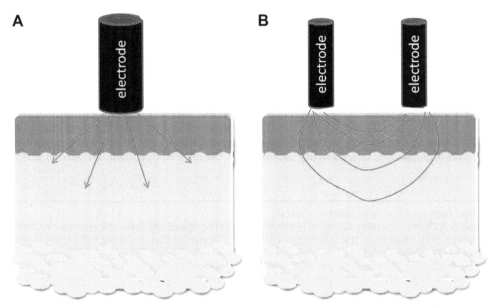

Fig. 2. Diagram demonstrating monopolar (*A*) and bipolar (*B*) electrode systems and their flow of electrical current through tissue. (*Adapted from* Bogle MA. Radiofrequency energy and hybrid devices. In: Alam M, Dover JS, editors. Procedures in cosmetic dermatology series: non-surgical skin tightening and lifting. Philadelphia: WB Saunders; 2008. p. 22; with permission.)

amounts of coupling fluid (ie, increased skin hydration) in certain radiofrequency procedures.[1]

Temperature also influences tissue conductivity. The distribution of electrical current within the skin can be influenced by preheating or cooling selected targets within the field. Every 1°C increase in temperature lowers the skin impedance by roughly 2%.[1] If one wants to increase the penetration depth of radiofrequency energy within the field, surface cooling can be used to increase resistance to the electrical field near the epidermis such that the current is driven deeper into the skin. Using the reverse line of thinking, it is possible to selectively increase the amount of radiofrequency energy that reaches a particular target in the skin by preheating it with optical energy from a laser. Prewarming a target, such as a hair or vessel, will, in theory, decrease resistance and increase conductivity of the radiofrequency current.[1]

MONOPOLAR RADIOFREQUENCY

The first device to use monopolar radiofrequency energy for skin tightening was the ThermaCool device (Thermage, Inc., Haywood, CA), introduced in 2001.[1] The ThermaCool device uses capacitive coupling to deliver radiofrequency energy to the skin through a thin membrane in the treatment tip. This unique system distributes the energy over a three-dimensional volume of skin, thereby delivering uniform heating at controlled depths to the deep dermis and subdermal layers of the skin to cause immediate collagen contraction and subsequent remodeling over the course of months.

Volumetric heating of the dermis is thought to lead to direct tissue tightening by breaking hydrogen bonds in the collagen triple helix, causing contraction.[1] This heat-induced collagen denaturation occurs at a threshold temperature of approximately 65°C.[6–8] Studies have also shown contraction of fibrous septa in the subcutaneous fat posttreatment, which is thought to be responsible for inward (Z-dimensional) tightening.[9] Collagen denaturation and contraction of the fibrous septa in the subcutaneous fat are thought to contribute to immediate, visible tightening the day of the procedure. Continued improvement over the course of 4 to 6 months is thought to derive from neocollagenesis and a delayed wound healing response.

Several pivotal clinical studies have been performed looking at treatment outcomes with monopolar radiofrequency.[1] Fitzpatrick and colleagues[10] studied monopolar radiofrequency for periorbital skin tightening using the original

1.0 cm³ Thermage treatment tips and found some degree of clinical improvement in 80% of subjects. Another trial using the 1.0 cm³ tips in the treatment of cheek, jawline, and neck laxity revealed softening of nasolabial and mesolabial folds in 28 of 30 subjects, with peak improvement of 35% to 40% 1 month posttreatment.[11] In the same study, improvement in submandibular and neck laxity was observed in 17 of 20 subjects, with peak improvement of 30% to 35% 3 months posttreatment.[11]

A split-face study analyzing changes to the brow and superior palpebral crease revealed an average 4.3 mm brow elevation and 1.9 mm superior palpebral crease elevation along the midpupillary line, and an average 2.4 mm brow elevation along the lateral canthal line.[12] The same study objectively measured jowl surface-area changes during split-face treatment of the cheek and found a mean decrease of 22.6% on the treated side indicating objective measurable tightening. No improvements were noted on the untreated side.[12]

Monopolar radiofrequency has also been studied for use in improving the appearance of cellulite. In a split-design study with 10 participants, one thigh was treated with up to six unilateral treatments at 2-week intervals while the other thigh served as a control.[13] While the data trended toward clinically visible and quantifiable improvement in dimple depth, density, and distribution, results did not achieve statistical significance.[13]

The BTC-2000 device (SRLI Technologies, Nashville, Tennessee) has been used to objectively measure skin elasticity and stiffness by extrapolating data from a stress strain curve.[14] In one study by Bogle and colleagues, monopolar radiofrequency treatments were performed on the lower face with the revised low-energy, multiple pass technique, and subjects were analyzed by total number of pulses delivered. Subjects with the highest number of pulses delivered (556) had an 80% increase in skin stiffness and an 80% improvement in elasticity. Subjects with a medium number of pulses (216) had a 74% improvement in stiffness and a 52% improvement in elasticity, while subjects with the lowest number of pulses (139) had only 26% improvement in stiffness and 33% improvement in elasticity.[14] This study was important in that it showed a definite correlation between the number of pulses delivered and the ability to achieve more consistent, predictable results.

A multicenter survey was conducted in 2006 to compare the original single-pass, high-energy technique with the revised low-energy, multiple-pass technique using immediate tissue tightening as a real-time endpoint.[15] With the original treatment algorithm, 26% of subjects saw immediate tightening and 54% observed skin tightening at 6 months. Almost half (45%) of the subjects thought the procedure was overly painful, and 68% found treatment results met their expectations. With the updated algorithm, 87% had immediate tissue tightening and 92% had some degree of tightening at 6 months, which was a significant increase in comparison with the previous results. Subjects found the updated protocol much less uncomfortable, with only 5% rating the procedure as overly painful, and satisfaction improved, with almost all subjects (94%) stating the procedure matched their expectations.[15] The low-energy, multiple-pass protocol also appears to be significantly safer, lowering the incidence of adverse events to less than 0.05% from the previous less than 1%.[16]

Monopolar radiofrequency has been established as safe for treatment of eyelid skin laxity using the ThermaCool 0.25 cm^3 shallow treatment tip at fluencies of 68 to 100 J/cm^2.[17] In one study, 87% of subjects showed at least 25% tightening of the upper lids and 67% showed at least 25% tightening of the lower lids with five passes using 12 to 14J.[18] Upper eyelids appear to respond more favorably than lower eyelids. Thirteen percent of upper eyelids and 33% of lower eyelids showed no improvement at 6 months. Despite these numbers, however, subjects were surprisingly more satisfied with their results on the lower eyelids than the upper eyelids.[18] One subject in the study had more passes than the others (8 versus 5), and this subject had the greatest degree of tightening, which again confirms the theory that subjects tend to do better with a higher number of passes.[14,18] All subjects must wear plastic corneoscleral protective lenses during eyelid treatments.

Generally, a single monopolar radiofrequency treatment is performed in a standard protocol.[1] Some patients may, however, gain some benefit from additional procedures. One study reported 80% of subjects achieved significant eyebrow lifting after four treatments compared with 60% after a single treatment.[19] Similarly, another study reported greater improvement in tightening of the nasolabial fold with two treatments spaced 1 month apart.[20] Patients could probably benefit from a touch-up treatment at some interval to help maintain results, however, the number of treatments for a specific individual should be discussed on a case by case basis.

The most common potential problems with radiofrequency skin tightening are discomfort during the procedure, temporary postoperative surface irregularities, postoperative changes in sensation, and unrealistic patient expectations. Most of these have been greatly reduced with the revised low-energy, multiple-pass treatment protocols. If needed, patients' pain can be controlled with topical, oral or intramuscular (IM) analgesics, however, it is best to just lower the treatment settings if patients are having pain. Postoperative surface irregularities or changes in sensation were more common with the original 1.0 cm^3 tips and are rare with the newer fast tips.[1] If patients do get surface irregularities, they are usually small nodules that are felt, but difficult to see, and self resolve in a few weeks. Changes in sensation may include itching or numbness. Symptoms are usually mild and resolve completely in days to weeks.

Rarely, side effects related to overly aggressive treatment may occur, such as burns, indentations, scars, or changes in pigmentation. These side effects are extremely unlikely to happen with the use of the newer tips and the low-energy, multiple-pass protocol.[1]

COMBINED ELECTRICAL AND OPTICAL ENERGY

Combined electrical and optical energy is another type of technology that uses radiofrequency energy and optical energy from laser or light sources within the same device. The radiofrequency component of the combined electrical and optical energy units currently available use bipolar electrodes rather than monopolar radiofrequency systems. This technology has shown efficacy in hair removal, wrinkle reduction, and the treatment of pigment and vascular disorders.[1]

There are several devices that use combined radiofrequency and laser or light technology including the Aurora, Polaris, and Galaxy systems (Syneron Medical Ltd., Yokneam, Israel). The Aurora combines radiofrequency and intense pulsed light in systems for hair removal, skin rejuvenation, and acne treatment. The Polaris combines radiofrequency and a 900 nm diode laser in systems for wrinkle reduction and vascular lesions. The Galaxy incorporates the Aurora and Polaris in a single device.

The advantage to this technology is that it takes advantage of the best of both worlds. For example, in skin rejuvenation, the laser component is able to address superficial lentigines and telangiectasias, while the radiofrequency component is theoretically able to penetrate deeper into the skin than standard nonablative lasers to induce thermal changes, limited to a depth of one half the distance between the bipolar electrodes.

For other indications, such as hair removal and the treatment of vascular lesions, the goal is to heat the target to a sufficient temperature that causes permanent injury. The combined forms of energy act synergistically to generate heat at the target. Target structures that have been preheated with optical energy, in theory, have greater conductivity, less resistance, and therefore should preferentially absorb the radiofrequency current administered after the optical pulse. With the combined radiofrequency and optical energy devices, there is an initial radiofrequency pulse delivered for calibration. This pulse is followed by pulses of optical and radiofrequency energy that are initiated at the same time. The radiofrequency pulse is then extended for a longer duration to take advantage of the greater conductivity in the heated tissue.[1]

A study evaluating bipolar radiofrequency combined with a 900 nm diode laser for the treatment of facial rhytides revealed more than half of participants had greater than 50% improvement in the appearance of wrinkles, and all reported at least some improvement in skin texture.[20,21] A second study of combined light and radiofrequency energy on photodamaged skin in a series of three to five treatments revealed a 70% improvement in facial redness and telangiectasias, a 78% improvement in lentigines, and a 60% improvement in skin texture.[22]

Combined optical and radiofrequency energy has also been studied in adult women with blond or white facial hair.[23] Subjects received four treatments 8 to 12 weeks apart using 15 to 30 J/cm^2 optical energy and 10 to 20 J/cm^3 radiofrequency energy. Results showed a hair clearance of 40% to 60%.[23] As with other technologies, hair removal efficacy appears to be greater in patients with darker hair (mean clearance 80% to 85%).[1,24]

Side effects associated with combined electrical-optical energy are uncommon. Because the two forms of energy act synergistically, lower levels of each can be used more effectively than when either component is used separately.[1] Lower-energy levels also allow patients to tolerate the procedure well with minimal discomfort and no need for adjunctive analgesics. The most common side effect is transient erythema immediately after the procedure, usually resolving in minutes to hours. Crusting, blisters, pigmentary change, and scarring are rare.

HYBRID MONOPOLAR AND BIPOLAR RADIOFREQUENCY

A hybrid radiofrequency system uses two hand pieces (one monopolar, one bipolar) (Accent RF, Alma Lasers, Ltd., Caesarea, Israel) to theoretically take advantage of two mechanisms of radiofrequency-induced tissue heating.[1] The monopolar hand piece achieves heating by way of the rotational movement of water molecules in the alternating current of the electromagnetic field to achieve volumetric heating at deeper levels in the skin (up to 20 mm).[25] The bipolar hand piece is used for superficial (2 to 6 mm), localized (nonvolumetric) heating based on tissue resistance to the radiofrequency conductive current.[6,25]

In a study looking at hybrid monopolar and bipolar radiofrequency treatments for the treatment of facial rhytides and skin laxity, 56% of participants had some degree of improvement in the appearance of rhytides and skin laxity. Out of 16 total women treated in the study, 12 had cheek treatments with five achieving 51% to 75% improvement and two achieving greater than 75% improvement.[6] Nine had jowl treatments with four achieving 51% to 75% improvement and one achieving greater than 75% improvement. Seven had periorbital treatments with three achieving 51% to 75% improvement, and eight had forehead treatments with three achieving 51% to 75% improvement.[6] Younger women (aged 25 to 45 years) had a higher satisfaction rate than older patients,[8] perhaps because the older group may have done better with adjunctive lifting procedures, such as fillers.[6]

Hybrid monopolar and bipolar radiofrequency treatments have also been studied for reduction of cellulite on the buttocks and thighs. Del Pino and colleagues[25] reported 68% of subjects achieved a 20% volumetric reduction of the subcutaneous adipose tissue after two treatment sessions.

The unipolar and bipolar hand pieces on a radiofrequency device have been compared in a split-face study for the treatment of facial rhytides and laxity.[26] Ten subjects received four treatments at 1-week intervals with approximately four passes of unipolar radiofrequency treatment on one side of the face and approximately four passes of bipolar radiofrequency treatment on the opposite side of the face. The degree of improvement approached, but did not achieve, statistical significance for either hand piece.[26]

As with the other radiofrequency devices, side effects are uncommon but may include burns, skin breakdown, or scarring with the use of inappropriately high energies.[1] As patients' discomfort tends to increase with higher energies, pain can be used as a feedback mechanism that the energy is too high. Operator technique is also important for optimal patient safety. The hand piece should be kept in motion when it is in contact with the skin to avoid areas of localized overheating and possible ulceration.[1] No instances of subcutaneous fat atrophy have been reported.

VACUUM-ASSISTED BIPOLAR RADIOFREQUENCY

Vacuum-assisted bipolar radiofrequency (Aluma, Lumenis Inc., Santa Clara, California) combines bipolar radiofrequency and vacuum technology in what has been called FACES technology (Functional Aspiration Controlled Electrothermal Stimulation). The device has a vacuum integrated in the hand piece that suctions a section of skin between two electrodes (**Fig. 3**). The purpose of this is to limit the volume of treated tissue to the skin between the electrodes and allow more specific treatment of targeted layers of the skin or subcutaneous fat with lower overall energy. Nontarget structures, such as muscle and bone, are avoided because they are not suctioned up between the electrodes.[1]

Mechanical stress on fibroblasts from the vacuum suction[2,27] and increased blood perfusion by way of exposure to the vacuum[2] may also lead to increased collagen formation and contribute to increased clinical efficacy; however, these theories remain to be clinically proven.

Gold and colleagues[2] studied vacuum-assisted bipolar radiofrequency in 46 adults with facial skin laxity. Study participants had eight treatments spaced 1 to 2 weeks apart. Using the Fitzpatrick-Goldman Classification of Wrinkling and Degree of Elastosis scale, the mean elastosis score went from 4.5 pretreatment to 2.5, 6 months posttreatment, with a general shift from moderate to mild elastosis. Researchers noted that although subjects were happy overall with the treatment outcome, satisfaction levels declined during the follow-up period.[2] This decline is thought to be a common finding in radiofrequency skin treatments because of delayed neocollagenesis and long-term wound healing response with small,

incremental changes.[1] Showing patients' baseline photography for comparison may help them more accurately remember their pretreatment skin condition and improve their overall satisfaction with the procedure.

Side effects that can rarely occur with vacuum-assisted bipolar-radiofrequency procedures include erythema, burns, blistering, edema, purpura, crusting, and transient hyperpigmentation.[2] Subcutaneous fat atrophy or indentations have not been reported.[1]

ULTRASOUND TECHNOLOGY

Intense, focused ultrasound has been used as a tool for the treatment of solid benign and malignant tumors for many decades, and is now emerging for tissue-tightening applications. As of early 2009, it is not yet approved for this indication by the US Food and Drug Administration. The primary mechanism of heat-induced tissue response by focused ultrasound shows coagulative necrosis with precisely defined, sharp margins caused by absorption of acoustic energy.[28] Ultrasound waves induce a vibration in the composite molecules of a given tissue during propagation, and the thermoviscous losses in the medium lead to tissue heating. The spectrum of cellular changes depends on the rise in temperature and the exposure duration and can range from total necrosis to more subtle ultrastructural cell damage with modulation of cellular cytokine expression.[28] These findings are similar to thermally induced changes in the skin after laser or light-induced heat applications.[29]

Intense focused ultrasound for skin-tightening applications uses short, millisecond pulses with a frequency in the megahertz domain, rather than kilohertz as is used in traditional high-intensity focused ultrasound (HIFU), to avoid cavitational processes. Another difference between intense

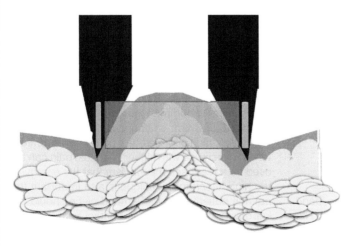

Fig. 3. In vacuum-assisted bipolar radiofrequency, skin is aspirated between two bipolar electrodes. (*Adapted from* Bogle MA. Radiofrequency energy and hybrid devices. In: Alam M, Dover JS, editors. Procedures in cosmetic dermatology series: non-surgical skin tightening and lifting. Philadelphia: WB Saunders; 2008. p. 24; with permission.)

focused ultrasound and traditional HIFU is that it uses significantly lower energies, 0.5 to 10J versus 100J, to allow thermal tissue changes without gross necrosis. The main advantages to focused ultrasound is that there is a potential for a greater depth of skin changes than other technologies are able to reach with the added benefit of precisely controlled, focal tissue injury. Experiments with a prototype device (Ulthera Inc., Mesa, Arizona) on postmortem skin show a focal depth of 4.2 mm below the skin surface.[29] This would potentially allow an external device to target traditionally surgical planes, such as the superficial muscular aponeurotic system (SMAS), for an enhanced tightening result.

Clinical evaluation of the Ulthera device has shown significant tightening with a 1-mm eyebrow lift 90 days posttreatment in more than 75% of study participants.[30] Minor side effects, such as redness and swelling, occurred following the procedure and resolved within a few hours.

PATIENT SELECTION

Nonsurgical skin tightening is best suited for patients with mild to moderate skin laxity without significant underlying structural ptosis. Patients with underlying laxity of the facial musculature, laxity of SMAS, or those with an excessive amount of skin laxity, are likely to have limited or no improvement with radiofrequency devices and should be counseled on other methods of rejuvenation including surgery.

The expected benefits of radiofrequency technology are controversial. The technology has shown benefit in the nasolabial folds, jowl, eyelid, brow, midface, jawline, and neck regions.[31] In addition, the technology has been used to tighten off-face areas, such as the thighs, arms, abdomen, and chest (**Fig. 4**).

Several studies have suggested that younger patients may respond better than older patients.[6,32] This is thought to occur because heat-labile collagen bonds are progressively replaced by irreducible multivalent cross links as the tissue ages, such that the skin of older individuals is less amenable to heat-induced tissue tightening.[32]

COMBINATION TREATMENT STRATEGY

Combination therapy is a dominant theme in cosmetic dermatology. Patients are able to achieve a more complete result when procedures, such as nonsurgical skin tightening, are combined with other therapies, such as botulinum toxin, fillers, and other modalities. Patients desiring a brow lift and more defined jawline may achieve additional benefit from the long-term adjunctive use of botulinum toxin to the superior-lateral orbicularis oculi and platysma muscles. Fillers can be used to achieve additional lift in the midface,

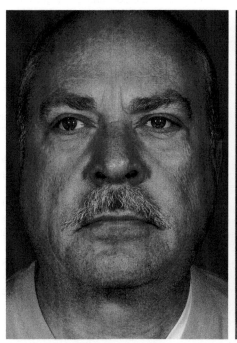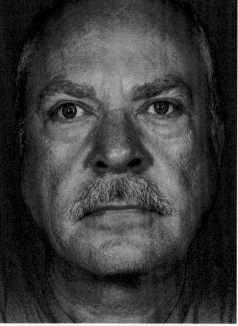

Fig. 4. Patient before (*left*) and 6 months after (*right*) monopolar radiofrequency treatment to the face and neck. Treatment by Marilyn Berzin, MD.(*Courtesy of* Thermage, Solta Medical, Hayward, CA; with permission.)

prejowl region, and jawline. Studies have shown monopolar radiofrequency skin tightening to be safe when performed over multiple soft-tissue fillers and may even have some synergistic effects in long-term collagen growth.[33]

SUMMARY

Results with current skin-tightening technologies are mild to moderate and are not intended to replace surgical procedures. Many patients will choose more subtle tightening to avoid the risks and downtime associated with surgery. Newer treatment protocols have improved treatment predictability and the extent of efficacy, and novel technologies, with the potential for even greater results, are currently in development. Overall patients' satisfaction can be increased by combining skin tightening with complementary, noninvasive skin treatments, such as botulinum toxin and soft-tissue fillers.

REFERENCES

1. Bogle MA. Radiofrequency energy and hybrid devices. In: Alam M, Dover JS, editors. Procedures in cosmetic dermatology series: non-surgical skin tightening and lifting. Philadelphia: WB Saunders; 2008. p. 21–32.
2. Gold MH, Goldman MP, Rao J, et al. Treatment of wrinkles and elastosis using vacuum-assisted bipolar radiofrequency heating of the dermis. Dermatol Surg 2007;33:300–9.
3. Sadick NS, Makino Y. Selective electro-thermolysis in aesthetic medicine: a review. Lasers Surg Med 2004;34:91–7.
4. Abraham MT, Ross EV. Current concepts in nonablative radiofrequency rejuvenation of the lower face and neck. Facial Plast Surg 2005;21:65–73.
5. Lack EB, Rachel JD, D'Andrea L, et al. Relationship of energy settings and impedance in different anatomic areas using a radiofrequency device. Dermatol Surg 2005;31:1668–70.
6. Friedman DJ, Gilead LT. The use of hybrid radiofrequency device for the treatment of rhytides and lax skin. Dermatol Surg 2007;33:543–51.
7. Mayoral FA. Skin tightening with a combined unipolar and bipolar radiofrequency device. J Drugs Dermatol 2007;6:212–5.
8. Zelickson B, Kist D, Bernstein E, et al. Histological and ultrastructural evaluation of the effects of a radiofrequency-based nonablative dermal remodeling device: a pilot study. Arch Dermatol 2004;140: 204–9.
9. Pope K, Levinson M, Ross EV. Selective fibrous tissue heating: an additional mechanism for capacitively coupled monopolar radiofrequency. Haywood, CA: Thermage, Inc; 2005.
10. Fitzpatrick R, Geronemus R, Goldberg D, et al. Multicenter study of noninvasive radiofrequency for periorbital tissue tightening. Lasers Surg Med 2003;33: 232–42.
11. Alster T, Tanzi E. Improvement of neck and cheek laxity with a nonablative radiofrequency device: a lifting experience. Dermatol Surg 2004;30:503–7.
12. Nahm WK, Su TT, Rotunda AM, et al. Objective changes in brow position, superior palpebral crease, peak angle of the eyebrow, and jowl surface area after volumetric radiofrequency treatments to half of the face. Dermatol Surg 2004;30:922–8.
13. Alexiades-Armenakas M, Dover JS, Arndt KA. Unipolar radiofrequency treatment to improve the appearance of cellulite. J Cosmet Laser Ther 2008; 10:148–53.
14. Bogle MA, Ubelhoer N, Weiss RA, et al. Evaluation of the multiple pass, low fluence algorithm for radiofrequency tightening of the lower face. Lasers Surg Med 2007;39:210–7.
15. Dover JS, Zelickson B, the 14-Physician multispecialty consensus panel. Results of a survey of 5,700 patient monopolar radiofrequency facial skin tightening treatments: assessment of a low-energy multiple-pass technique leading to a clinical end point algorithm. Dermatol Surg 2007;33:900–7.
16. Narins RS, Tope WD, Pope K, et al. Overtreatment effects associated with a radiofrequency tissue-tightening device: rare, preventable, and correctable with subcision and autologous fat transfer. Dermatol Surg 2006;32:115–24.
17. Biesman BS, Pope K. Monopolar radiofrequency treatment of the eyelids: a safety evaluation. Dermatol Surg 2007;33:794–801.
18. Carruthers J, Carruthers A. Shrinking upper and lower eyelid skin laxity with a novel radiofrequency tip. Dermatol Surg 2007;33:802–9.
19. Koch RJ. Radiofrequency nonablative tissue tightening. Facial Plast Surg Clin North Am 2004;12: 339–46.
20. Fritz M, Counters JT, Zelickson BD. Radiofrequency treatment for middle and lower face laxity. Arch Facial Plast Surg 2004;6:370–3.
21. Sadick NS, Trelles MA. Nonablative wrinkle treatment of the face and neck using a combined diode laser and radiofrequency technology. Dermatol Surg 2005;31:1695–9.
22. Bitter P Jr, Mulholland RS. Report of a new technique for enhanced non-invasive skin rejuvenation using a dual mode pulsed light and radiofrequency energy source: selective radiothermolysis. J Cosmet Dermatol 2002;1:142–5.
23. Sadick NS, Laughlin SA. Effective epilation of white and blond hair using combined radiofrequency and optical energy. J Cosmet Laser Ther 2004;6:27–31.

24. Sadick NS, Shaoul J. Hair removal using a combination of conducted radiofrequency and optical energies—an 18-month follow-up. J Cosmet Laser Ther 2004;6:21–6.

25. Del Pino E, Rosado RH, Azuela A, et al. Effect of controlled volumetric tissue heating with radiofrequency on cellulite and the subcutaneous tissue of the buttocks and thighs. J Drugs Dermatol 2006;5: 714–22.

26. Alexiades-Armenakas M, Dover JS, Arndt KA. Unipolar versus bipolar radiofrequency treatment of rhytides and laxity using a mobile painless delivery method. Lasers Surg Med 2008;40:446–53.

27. Eastwood M, McGrouther DA, Brown RA. Fibroblast responses to mechanical forces. Proc Inst Mech Eng 1998;212:85–92.

28. Van Leenders GJ, Beerlage HP, Ruijter ET, et al. Histopathological changes associated with high intensity focused ultrasound (HIFU) treatment for localized adenocarcinoma of the prostate. J Clin Pathol 2000;53:391–4.

29. Lauback HJ, Makin IRS, Barthe PG, et al. Intense focused ultrasound: evaluation of a new treatment modality for precise microcoagulation within the skin. Dermatol Surg 2008;34:727–34.

30. Alam M, White L, Majzoub R, et al. Safety and efficacy of transcutaneous ultrasound for forehead, cheek and neck tissue tightening. Lasers Surg Med 2007;S19:19.

31. Dierickx C. The role of deep heating for noninvasive skin rejuvenation. Lasers Surg Med 2006;38:799–807.

32. Hsu TS, Kaminer MS. The use of nonablative radiofrequency technology to tighten the lower face and neck. Semin Cutan Med Surg 2003;22:115–23.

33. Shumaker PR, England LJ, Dover JS, et al. Effect of monopolar radiofrequency treatment over soft-tissue fillers in an animal model: part 2. Lasers Surg Med 2006;38(3):211–7.

Cosmetic Dermatology: Legal Issues

David J. Goldberg, MD, JD[a,b,c,]*

KEYWORDS
- Cosmetic dermatology • Malpractice • Physician extenders
- Legal issues • Cosmeceuticals

Cosmetic dermatology is a continuously evolving field of medicine. According to the American Society for Dermatologic Surgery, in 2008, $13.2 billion was spent on cosmetic procedures and 82% of that amount went toward non-surgical techniques. According to the American Society for Aesthetic and Plastic Surgery, its members performed over 8 million non-invasive cosmetic procedures in 2008. The total number of these procedures is probably even higher. Laser and light-based procedures, fillers, toxins, and various peels have revolutionized the field of cosmetic dermatology. With an increasing number of physicians and nonphysicians performing these procedures, and with a seemingly unlimited array of cosmetic dermatology procedures, the potential for problems and their legal consequences continues to increase. This article discusses the concept of negligence and the potential for medical malpractice that may arise in this situation, including the associated problems that may arise when these procedures are performed by physician extenders. An understanding of the basic principals of a cause of action in medical malpractice may protect a physician from losing a malpractice suit. The impact of the physician and physician extender relationship, and the legal issues that arise from this relationship, are also discussed. The article concludes with the legal and ethical issues associated with the promotion of cosmeceutical agents in the field of cosmetic dermatology.

Although legal concerns can arise in the performance of any medical procedure, they are of increasing concern in the field of cosmetic dermatology. Most of the legal issues that arise in this context are in the realm of negligence.

Any analysis of physician negligence must first begin with a legal description of the elements of negligence. There are four required elements for a cause of action in negligence. They are duty, breach of duty, causation, and damages. The suing plaintiff must show the presence of all four elements to be successful in her claim.[1]

The duty of a physician performing cosmetic dermatology is to perform the cutaneous laser procedure in accordance with the standard of care. By extension of this principle, any employed physician extender performing cosmetic dermatology procedures under the direct supervision of a dermatologist will likely be held to the same standard as the physician. Although the elements of a cause of action in negligence are derived from formal legal textbooks, the standard of care is not necessarily derived from some well-known textbook. It is also not articulated by any judge. The standard of care is defined by some judges as whatever an expert witness says it is and what a jury will believe. In a case against any physician performing procedures in the field of cosmetic dermatology, the specialist must have and use the knowledge and skill ordinarily possessed by a specialist in that field under similar circumstances. A dermatologist, physician extender, or, for that matter, an internist practicing cosmetic dermatology will be held to an equal standard. A failure to fulfill such a duty may lead to that individual losing a lawsuit. If the jury accepts the suggestion that the provider mismanaged the case and that the negligence led to damage of the patient, then liability will ensue. Conversely, if the jury believes an expert

a Skin Laser & Surgery Specialists of New York and New Jersey, New York, NY, USA
b Mount Sinai School of Medicine, New York, NY, USA
c Fordham University School of Law, New York, NY, USA
* Corresponding author. Skin Laser & Surgery Specialists of New York and New Jersey, 115 E. 57th Street, Suite 710, New York, NY 10022, USA.
E-mail address: drdavidgoldberg@skinandlasers.com

Dermatol Clin 27 (2009) 501–505
doi:10.1016/j.det.2009.08.002
0733-8635/09/$ – see front matter © 2009 Elsevier Inc. All rights reserved.

who testifies for a defendant doctor, then the standard of care in that particular case has been met. In this view, the standard of care is a pragmatic concept, decided case by case, and based on the testimony of an expert physician. The sued physician or nonphysician is expected to perform the procedure in a manner of a reasonable physician. He need not be the best in his field; he need only perform the procedure in a manner that is considered by an objective standard as reasonable.

It is important to note that where there are two or more recognized methods of diagnosing or treating the same condition. A physician does not fall below the standard of care by using any of the acceptable methods, even if one method turns out to be less effective than another method. Finally, in many jurisdictions, an unfavorable result due to an physician's "error in judgment" by a physician is not in and of itself a violation of the standard of care if the physician acted appropriately before exercising his professional judgment.

Evidence of the standard of care in a specific malpractice case includes laws, regulations, and guidelines for practice (which represent a consensus among professionals on a topic involving diagnosis or treatment); and the medical literature, including peer-reviewed articles and authoritative texts. In addition, the view of an expert is crucial. Although the standard of care may vary from state to state, it is typically defined as a national standard by the profession at large.

Usually, for litigation purposes, an expert witness articulates the standard of care. The expert witness's testimony and the basis of the standard of care are grounded in the one or a combination of the following:

1. The witness's personal practice
2. Observation of practice of others
3. Medical literature in recognized publications
4. Statutes or legislative rules
5. Courses in which the subject is discussed and taught in a well-defined manner.

The standard of care is based on the way in which the majority of the physicians in a similar medical community practice. In this case, it is the method by which other laser physicians perform cosmetic dermatology. If the expert herself does not practice like the same way as the majority of other physicians, then the expert will have a difficult time explaining why the majority of the medical community has different practices.

It would seem that, in a perfect world, the standard of care in every case would be a clearly definable level of care agreed on by all physicians and patients. Unfortunately, in the typical situation the standard of care is an ephemeral concept resulting from differences and inconsistencies between the medical profession, the legal system, and the public.

At one extreme, the medical profession is dominant in determining the standard of care in the practice of medicine. Recommendations, guidelines, and policies regarding varying treatment modalities for different clinical situations published by nationally recognized boards, societies, and commissions establish the appropriate standard of care. In some of these cases, however, factual disputes may arise because different organizations will publish conflicting standards concerning the same medical condition. Adding to the confusion, local societies may publish their own rules applicable to a particular claim of malpractice.

Thus, in most situations, the standard of care is neither clearly definable nor consistently defined. It is a legal fiction to suggest that a generally accepted standard of care exists for any area of practice. At best, there are parameters within which experts will testify. Unfortunately, because of the increased acceptance of cosmetic dermatology—and unrealistic expectations by the public—physicians sometimes run the risk of being held to an unrealistic and unattainable standard of care. But, in the end Ultimately, the physician community establishes that standard of care. For example, most physicians suggest that the safest technique for the removal of unwanted hair is by use of the neodymium:yttrium-aluminum-garnet (Nd:YAG) laser. However, a physician using a non-Nd:YAG laser or light source that is also approved by the US Food and Drug Administration (FDA) for the treatment of unwanted hair in darker skin types may be performing laser treatment within the standard of care.

In recent years, physicians in the United States have put substantial efforts toward setting standards (ie, specifying treatment approaches to various conditions). Clinical practice guidelines, position statements, and practice guidelines have been developed by specialty societies such as the American Academy of Dermatology, the American Society for Dermatologic Surgery, and the American Society for Lasers in Medicine and Surgery.. These guidelines as they pertain to both cosmetic dermatology stipulate who can and who cannot perform various treatments, and in what settings nonphysicians can use cutaneous lasers. The Institute of Medicine has defined clinical guidelines as "systemically developed statements to assist practitioner and patient decisions about appropriate health care for specific clinical circumstances."[2] These guidelines represent standardized specifications for performing a procedure or managing a particular clinical problem.

Such clinical guidelines raise thorny legal issues.[3] They have the potential to offer an authoritative and settled statement of what the standard of care should be for a given treatable condition. Although they do not represent law, a judge would have several options when guidelines are offered as evidence. Such a guideline might be evidence of the customary practice in the medical profession. A dermatologist, or a physician extender working for that dermatologist, acting in accordance with the guidelines would be shielded from liability to the same extent as one who can establish that she or he followed professional customs. The guidelines could play the role of an authoritative expert witness or a well-accepted review article. However, using guidelines as evidence of professional custom is problematic if they are not consistent with prevailing medical practice. This is a common problem in the field of cosmetic dermatology since many members have chosen not to follow their professional society guidelines.

According to surveys of malpractice lawyers, clinical guidelines have already had an effect. A widely accepted clinical standard may be presumptive evidence of due care, but expert testimony will still be required to introduce the standard and establish its sources and relevancy.

Professional societies often attach disclaimers to their guidelines, thereby undercutting their use in litigation. The American Medical Association (AMA), for example, calls its guidelines parameters instead of protocols. This is intended to significantly impact on physician discretion. The AMA further suggests that all such guidelines contain disclaimers stating that they are not intended to replace physician discretion. Such guidelines cannot be treated as conclusive.

Usually, plaintiffs will use their own expert, as opposed to the physician's expert, to define the standard of care. Although a plaintiff's expert may also refer to clinical practice guidelines, the physician's negligence can be established in other ways. These methods include (1) examination of the physician defendant's expert witness; (2) an admission by the defendant that he or she was negligent; (3) testimony by the plaintiff, in the rare case where he or she is a medical expert qualified to evaluate the allegedly negligent physician's conduct; and (4) common knowledge in situations where a layperson could understand the negligence without the assistance of an expert.[4,5]

Rarely, cosmetic dermatology practices are located within hospitals or certified ambulatory care centers. In such situations, a plaintiff may seek hospital committee proceeding minutes pertaining to the allegedly negligent physician. The plaintiff may request that the committee produce its minutes or reports; set forth interrogatories about the committee process or outcome; or seek to depose committee members. If the plaintiff is suing a cosmetic dermatologist whose work was reviewed by the committee, the discovery process may seek to confirm the negligence of the professional or to uncover additional evidence substantiating the plaintiff's claims. Discovery requests are often met with a claim that information that is generated within or by a hospital committee is not discoverable. Judges have ruled that the discovery protection granted hospital quality-review committee records prevents the opposing party from taking advantage of a hospital's careful self-assessment.[6] The suing plaintiff must use his or her own experts to evaluate the facts underlying the incident. Some judges believe that immunity of committee proceedings protects certain communications and encourages the quality-review process. They argue that external access to committee investigations stifles candor and inhibits the constructive criticism thought necessary for a quality-review process. Constructive, objective, peer criticism might not occur because of apprehension that a physician's comments will be used in a malpractice suit as a denunciation of a colleague's conduct.

When a plaintiff seeks discovery of a facility or hospital incident report, rather than a committee proceeding, policy considerations are somewhat different. Incident reports kept in the medical records and possibly filed by a staff member are often more directly related to a single claim for malpractice than are general committee investigations. Judges are usually less willing to protect such incident reports.

Because the field of cosmetic dermatology has evolved rapidly over the past decade, physicians are quick to try innovations and experimental concepts. Such innovations partially explain the excitement of this growing field. New laser surgical procedures and the treatment of conditions that were once untreatable (ie, port-wine stains and nevus of Ota) may fall into regulatory gaps not covered by the strict regulations for the laser device itself. Licensing through the FDA carefully regulates medical devices such as lasers.[7] However, a variety of dermal fillers and botulinum toxin are off-label and not cleared by the FDA.

Such experimentation is one reason for the explosive growth of cosmetic dermatology. Most human experimentation is governed by regulations of the US Department of Health and Human Services. The regulations require that an institution sponsoring research must establish an institutional review board. The board evaluates research proposals before any experimentation begins in order to determine whether human subjects might be at risk and, if so, how to protect them.

It is not usually difficult to determine whether a new cosmetic dermatologic procedure is being used experimentally. It is, however, very difficult to determine whether an actual procedure is experimental. Cosmetic dermatologists often view themselves not as experimenters, but as artists and scientists customizing a treatment for a particular condition. Such approaches can lead to a bad result with variable outcomes in the courts. A dermatologist using a standard laser hair-removal system around the eyelashes with resultant damage to the iris will be questioned. A laser surgeon who chooses to use a carbon dioxide laser, rather than a scalpel, to perform a circumcision procedure, with a resultant complication leading to penile amputation would have problems suggesting that his or her medical experimentation conformed to reasonable standard of care. However, if another dermatologist chooses (after appropriate informed consent) to use the same laser (rather than a scalpel) for excision of a nevus, and no significant scarring results, she or he might be considered an innovator rather than an experimenter. A dermatologist trying botulinum toxin for hair growth or as filler for penile enhancement might also be seen as an innovator. Such aThis physician would be no more liable for straying from his or her duty than the physician who uses a standard procedure resulting in the same complication.

In fact, most clinical innovation falls between standard practice and experimental research. Much of this innovation is unregulated by the government. The National Commission for the Protection of Human Subjects of Biomedical and Behavioral Research has suggested that any "radically new" procedure should be made the object of formal research at an early stage to determine whether such a procedure is safe and effective.[8] It can be argued that some of the cosmetic dermatology procedures that have evolved using already FDA-cleared devices or drugs might be considered radical; clearly, most are not.

It is apparent that, in order for the plaintiff to win a negligence cause of action against the cosmetic dermatologist, he or she must establish that the physician had a duty of reasonable care and had breached that duty. However, that breach must lead to some form of damage. A mere inconvenience to the plaintiff, even in the event of a physician's breach, will usually not lead to physician liability.

These issues become magnified when the procedure is performed by a physician extender. Who can perform those procedures is governed by state law—not by any specialty society. Laws vary from state to state and will always outweigh a more liberal society guideline. Where the nonphysician is legally performing laser treatments, and is performing within the scope of his or her duty, both the physician extender and the physician will be found liable for the negligence.

An increasingly popular aspect of the cosmetic dermatology practice is the sale of various cosmeceutical products. Products with "Dr" or "MD" on the label, or those known to be manufactured by a physician under an innocuous logo, are easy to find. The appeal of creating such products is obvious: the rewards are great. Sales of these products will possibly lead to tens of millions of dollars in gross revenue; a Madison Avenue store; and the power, access, and prestige associated with such products. Dermatologists enter this market because they offer what sells. There are no gastroenterologists selling fiber-fortified cereals, bottling their own brand of water, or patenting a superior stool softener. The market is just not there. There is nothing inherently wrong with creating a product. It is especially worthwhile if a cosmetic dermatologist offers a uniquely effective topical agent. Consumers may believe that an "MD" brand is better, more helpful, really is different, and that the cosmetic dermatologist aims to help patients, not exploit them. The problem is that physician-sold cosmeceuticals may not be more potent than other readily available products. Although some dermatologists engaging in these ventures claim years of research and clinical trials, their claims may be as unsubstantiated as those of cosmetic companies. Assertions are not scientific proof. Some patients may suspect physicians who recommend their own scientifically unproven product. They may be well-informed enough to separate medical dermatology from skin-care panaceas, even though they are offered in the same office. In addition, they may resist the social pressure to buy their physician's product. Then again, they may not. It becomes ethically suspect, breaching obligations of beneficence and honesty (among others), when cosmetic dermatologists trade on their status to sell a clinically unproven product. Using the power of a medical degree as a marketing tool may be shrewd, but it is unethical if the product cannot withstand scientific scrutiny. Cosmetics companies may be able to duck the issue of truth in advertising, but they are not bound by the same ethical obligations as physicians. Physicians who make and sell their own products may become self-interested, although they should adhere to a high standard and prove the efficacy of what they sell. It is better to have an in-office esthetician marketing these products than the dermatologist him- or herself. However, if a patient is hurt by a product, the medical malpractice issues become that much more obvious.

A variety of legal and ethical issues can arise within the cosmetic dermatology practice. Usually these relate to issues of medical malpractice. It is often difficult to predict the outcome in a malpractice cause of action against a dermatologist. However, a clear understanding of the aforementioned principles will markedly decrease the chance of a physician losing any negligence cause of action brought against him or her.

REFERENCES

1. Furrow BF, Greaney TL, Johnson SH, et al. Liability in health care law. 3rd edition. St. Paul (MN): West Publishing Co; 1997.
2. Lohr KM, Field MJ. Guidelines for Clinical Practice. Washington, DC: The National Academies Press; 1992.
3. Hyams AL, Shapiro DW, Brennan TA. Medical practice guidelines in malpractice litigation: an early retrospective. J Health Polit Policy Law 1996;289–98.
4. Lamont v. Brookwood Health Service, Inc., 446 So.2d 1018 (Ala.1983).
5. Gannon v. Elliot, 19 Cal.App.4th 1 (1993).
6. Coburn v. Seda, 101 Wash.2d 270 (1984).
7. Federal Food, Drug, and Cosmetic Act, 21 U.S.C.A. s301.
8. National Research Act, Pub L 93:348.

Complications and Their Management in Cosmetic Dermatology

Ranella Hirsch, MD, FAAD*, Meghan Stier, BS

KEYWORDS

- Cosmetic complication • Botox
- Dermatology • Restylane • Juvederm

More cosmetic dermatologic rejuvenation options exist today than ever before; however, as with all medical procedures, these treatments carry attendant risk. This article examines the risks of popular nonsurgical cosmetic rejuvenation options and the best treatment options should complications occur.

PATIENT SCREENING AND SELECTION

An initial patient intake interview should begin with a series of open-ended questions to determine what areas are of greatest concern to a patient. It is critical that patients are given realistic expectations regarding results and potential complications. Patients typically arrive for a consultation with some understanding of cosmetic rejuvenation but a physician often needs to address any misperceptions.

Patients should be asked about their medical history, including, but not limited to, a history of keloids, scarring, clotting disorders, and cold sores. The herpes simplex virus (HSV) infection can be reactivated with some procedures. As this increases the risk of dyspigmentation or scarring, standard practice is to prescribe prophylactic, valacyclovir, beginning 2 to 3 days preprocedure in patients at risk.[1]

CHEMICAL PEEL COMPLICATIONS

Chemical peels have been used safely in cosmetic dermatology to excellent effect for decades. Chemical peels are classified as superficial, medium, or deep. Superficial peels can be performed at a physician's office with resorcinol or 10% to 35% trichloracetic acid (TCA), whereas other agents are for at-home use (tretinoin, salicylic acid, α-hydroxy acids, and 5-fluorouracil).[2] Medium peel agents include Jessner's solution (lactic acid, salicylic acid, and resorcinol in ethyl alcohol, all 14% weight to volume), a combination of Jessner's solution and 35% TCA, 70% glycolic acid, a combination of 70% glycolic acid and 35% TCA, and a combination of CO_2 and 35% TCA.[2–4] For the most significant peeling, TCA concentration must reach at least 35%, although if the solution is too concentrated (TCA 40% or higher), patients are at greater risk for scarring.[4] Deep peels generally used the Baker-Gordon phenol solution, a mixture of 50% to 55% phenol, liquid soap (Septisol), and croton oil, and are rarely performed.

Peels are contraindicated in patients who cannot avoid sunlight, patients who cannot use cosmetic cover-up,[5] patients with a history of previous isotretinoin or irradiation treatment, patients who smoke, patients taking immunosuppressive medications, or patients with a history of HSV or hypertrophic scarring.[5] Complications are also more likely to occur in patients with metabolic problems that delay wound healing, such as diabetes mellitus, cardiovascular disease, and lupus erythematous, or in patients who are not psychologically prepared for the downtime that follows treatment.[4]

Skincare Doctors, 777 Concord Avenue, Suite 206, Cambridge, MA 02138, USA
* Corresponding author.
E-mail address: ranella@skincaredoctors.com (R. Hirsch).

Dermatol Clin 27 (2009) 507–520
doi:10.1016/j.det.2009.08.013
0733-8635/09/$ – see front matter © 2009 Published by Elsevier Inc.

Common, Transient Complications

Pruritus is common during the re-epithelialization process and can last up to 1 month. Agents used to treat erythema, including topical hydrocortisone (2.5%), oral antihistamines, and short-term systemic steroids, may help. Pruritus with slow healing, increased erythema, or follicular pustules on the neck or outside of the peel region may signal contact dermatitis, which can be treated with hydrocortisone creams and antihistamines as needed.[5] It is expected that mid- to deep-level peels produce edema, erythema, and desquamation, and patients should be educated about this possibility during the informed consent process.[3]

Significant Side Effects

Allergic reaction

Dermal peels can cause allergic reactions but these may be difficult to diagnose. The symptoms of an allergic reaction to the peel can be strikingly similar to those caused by the peel itself and include erythema, edema, pruritus, burning, and stinging. These reactions may manifest as contact dermatitis or cold, cholinergic, or contact urticaria.[2] In general, physicians may suspect an allergic reaction if patients develop erythema and edema on nonpeeled areas, if urticaria appears on the body, if there is serious itching or edema only a few hours after the peel, or if patients have trouble breathing and experience throat constriction.[6] Patients should also be instructed to avoid potential contact sensitizers, such as neomycin, aloe vera, and vitamin E.[2]

Allergic contact reactions occur most frequently with resorcinol.[2] In addition, salicylic acid, which is used in superficial peels and in Jessner's solution, may rarely lead to systemic toxicity from salicylates, otherwise known as salicylism. Symptoms can present when plasmic salicylic acid levels are as low as 10 to 35 mg/100 mL.[2] Given the limited area for peels, patient risk for salicylism is extremely low, unless peeling is expanded to include simultaneous treatment of several other regions (such as the chest, arms, and legs), a practice that is contraindicated. Salicylic acid may also cause contact urticaria.[2]

Acne and milia

The development of acne during healing or after re-epithelialization can range from pustular to cystic, and a previous history of acne is not always established, although recent tretinoin use before the peel or greasy moisturizers applied after the peel may exacerbate the problem.[5] Postpeel acne can be treated with topical and oral antibiotics. To minimize the development of scars that may occur with cystic acne, patients may be treated with intralesional triamcinolone acetonide and a rapidly tapering course of prednisone for 1 week.[5]

Milia may also appear 2 to 3 weeks after re-epithelialization and may be triggered by the use of thick ointments.[5] Patients should be aware that milia may also result as a normal part of neocollagenesis. Milia may be treated with gentle epidermabrasion after re-epithelialization, topical tretinoin before and after the peel, electrodesiccation, or extraction with a #11 scalpel blade.[5]

Delayed wound healing

Wound healing that is slower than anticipated and prolonged erythema are indications that peeled skin is healing abnormally. Delayed healing from medium peels presents by day 8 and by days 10 to 14 after deep peels.[5] Delayed healing is defined as the appearance of friable, stellate, nonindurated unhealed erosions with serous granulation tissue at the expected final days of healing. Often, there can be no indication during the peel process that aberrant re-epithelialization will occur.[5] These erosions may heal with hypopigmented, flat scarring. Artificial wound dressings (Vigilon, Bard Medical, Covington, Georgia) can facilitate the wound healing process and reduce healing time.[3,5]

Persistent erythema is defined as prolonged if it lasts longer than 3 to 5 days for a superficial peel, 15 to 30 days for a midlevel peel, or 90 days for a deep peel.[7] Such erythema can be treated with topical hydrocortisone lotion (2.5%), oral antihistamines, short-term systemic steroids, or silicone gel sheeting, depending on the degree of presentation.[5]

Delayed wound healing and extended erythema are often harbingers of bacterial (or, more rarely, fungal) infection, and cultures should be taken. Empiric antibiotics are appropriate for initial management and then anti-infective treatment can be tailored to the specific pathogen.

Periorbital peels and forehead peels can cause significant edema, especially in the orbital region. In some cases, this swelling may be enough to shut the eyelids.[3]

Infection

Bacterial, viral, or candidal infections occur early in the healing stage and first present as delayed areas of wound healing, ulcerations, granulation tissue lasting more than 7 to 10 days, or an accumulation of necrotic tissue with disproportionate scabbing, crusting, purulent drainage, and odor.[3] Clinicians must remain highly attuned to post-treatment care as infections may just initially present as erythema.

Bacterial infections can appear in the first 3 to 10 days after the procedure, although some infections can occur several weeks post peel.[8] This risk is greatly lessened with appropriate antibiotic prophylaxis. Viral reactivations occur within the first 7 to 10 days before re-epithelialization. If patients are taking antiviral medication, reactivation can occur immediately after finishing antiviral therapy, particularly if the dose is too low or the course is too short.[8] Yeast infections generally appear later than bacterial or viral infections, usually surfacing between days 9 and 17 post procedure.[9]

Infectious complications can include toxic shock syndrome (the most severe complication), HSV reactivation, candidiasis, bacterial pyoderma, and Epstein-Barr virus keratitis.[5] Patients with HSV should be particularly cautious about chemical peels, as postoperative problems may carry substantial morbidity.[3]

Cultures should be taken when necessary and after a diagnosis is made, infections should be treated with the appropriate antimicrobial agent. Dilute vinegar soaks post treatment can also help reduce the risk of infection.[4] All patients receiving medium to deep peels, regardless of HSV status, should also receive prophylactic oral antivirals starting the day before treatment and continuing for 5 days postoperatively (10 to 14 days postoperatively for HSV patients).[3,7,10] Patients with a history of frequent HSV outbreaks should receive prophylaxis even before superficial peels.[7]

Scarring
Although persistent erythema is often a sign of delayed healing, it may also be an early sign of scarring, and aggressive treatment in such cases is imperative. Early administration of medium- to high-potency topical steroids is recommended, and steroid-impregnated tape (Cordran Tape, Oclassen Pharmaceuticals, Morristown, New Jersey) and silicone gel sheeting may also be helpful. Pulsed dye laser treatment every 6 to 8 weeks can improve scarring by as much as 50% after two treatments. Intralesional triamcinolone may follow if necessary.[4,5,11] Patients with darker skin tones (phototypes III–VI) carry a greater risk of hypertrophic scars or keloids after any cutaneous trauma.[12] Keloids are a particular risk for patients of African, Spanish, or Asian origin,[13] and keloid formation may be influenced by genetics,[14,15] In addition, smoking, inadequate topical hydration, constrictive taping, and infections may all contribute to the risk of scarring.[5]

Dyschromias
Medium and deep peels can carry a serious risk of post-treatment pigmentary problems. Patients with skin types III to VI, patients with excessive sun exposure, and patients with preoperative pigmentary problems (melasma or postinflammatory hyperpigmentation) are at greatest risk.[4]

Hyperpigmentation usually appears 3 to 4 weeks post peel and, like hypopigmentation, is especially common in patients with previous pigmentary issues or darker Fitzpatrick skin phototypes. It is also more prevalent in patients who use birth control pills, exogenous estrogens, or photosensitizing drugs or in patients who become pregnant within 6 months of the peel.[5] Hyperpigmentation can be managed with hydroquinones and low-potency topical steroids.[4]

Hypopigmentation is a highly undesired outcome of chemical peeling and is generally permanent. A line of demarcation may occur wherever the peel stops, and this can be particularly problematic for patients with darker skin or freckles.[4] Feathering, or applying solutions approximately 5 mm past the borders of the indicated area, may decrease visibility of the demarcation line.[5] Hypopigmentation may occur in patients who undergo deep peeling the in the perioral or periorbital areas alone, and this is generally considered a conspicuous deformity. To provide a more uniform appearance, the remaining areas of the face should be treated with a medium-depth peel.[3]

LASER AND LIGHT DEVICE COMPLICATIONS

Laser therapies fall into three main categories: nonablative resurfacing, fractional resurfacing, and ablative resurfacing. Nonablative technologies include intense pulsed light; infrared lasers; photodynamic therapy; vascular lasers, such as the pulsed dye laser; radiofrequency devices; and some fractional resurfacing lasers. Ablative lasers, such as the CO_2 and Er:YAG devices, remain the gold standards of rejuvenation for photodamaged skin but carry a more significant risk of side effects (dyspigmentation, scarring, and textural changes) and require patients willing to tolerate a prolonged recovery phase.[10] Fractional ablative lasers can be an effective alternative to traditional ablative lasers and carry a lower yield of total side effects.[16]

Common, Transient Complications

Transient purpura, crusting, or edema may occur after any laser treatment. Use of adequate epidermal protection and the lowest effective energy settings minimize these common complications.[17]

Cooling Device Damage

Skin cooling during laser treatment increases patient safety and improves results by limiting the extent of epidermal damage. If skin cooling devices malfunction or are improperly used, patients are at greater risk for thermal injury. The inconsistent application of aluminum rollers, failure of water chilling, inadequate beam contact, retrograde motion of copper tips, or bubbles in the line between the cryogen canister and laser hand piece may lead to insufficient cooling, increased pain, and unwanted tissue reactions.[17] Treating physicians must be familiar with the specific device and use the appropriate precooling, parallel cooling, and postcooling methods. Physicians should also take care to determine the best duration of cryogen spray for the device's parameters and increase fluences slowly as cooling begins. To ensure cooling is adequate, it is important to test the cooled tip before starting therapy and to pay close attention to a patient's pain response and the appearance of cutaneous surface color immediately post treatment.[17]

Significant Side Effects

Textural changes

In rarely reported cases,[17,18] patients may show no initial evidence of epidermal injury only to develop textural changes 1 to 2 months after treatment if deeper tissues were overheated during their procedures.[18] Such depressions may resolve after 6 to 10 months, or infrared or visible light lasers can be used for nonablative dermal remodeling.[17] Narins and colleagues[18] advise subcision with autologous fat transfer to correct depressions lasting for more than 6 months caused by radiofrequency devices.

To prevent contour irregularities, physicians should use the most appropriate conservative fluences, judiciously perform test spots, allow for pauses between passes, and follow a treatment grid to avoid overlap when necessary. Although patient comfort is paramount, aggressive pain management during treatment should be avoided, as patient sensations are an important source of feedback for clinicians and can be a critical early warning sign of overtreatment.[18]

Acne and milia

Acne and milia are most likely caused by post-treatment dressings and ointments and disruption of follicular units during treatment and re-epithialization. Acne can be treated with retinoids, a short course of oral antibiotics, or topical antibiotics if the skin has completely re-epithelialized. Milia may be treated with retinoic acid or manual extraction.[19,20]

Allergic reaction

Eczematous dermatitis may develop during the first 4 weeks post operation and responds to the proper use of emollients and topical midpotency corticosteroids. Perioral dermatitis is rarely seen in the first 3 months after treatment and is best managed with a course of oral doxycycline. Irritant contact dermatitis may also occur due to topical anesthetics and may resolve by treatment with topical or oral corticosteroids.[10]

Dyschromias

The risk of pigmentary change is linked to the depth of laser damage. Injury in the papillary dermis typically leads to temporary postinflammatory hyperpigmentation, whereas deeper injury can cause permanent hypopigmentation.[10] Patients with Fitzpatrick skin phototypes III to VI are especially prone to pigmentary problems post treatment. As with textural changes, pigmentary problems can often be avoided with improved physician technique and vigorous patient compliance with aftercare.[18]

Hyperpigmentation develops within the first month post treatment and usually resolves spontaneously within subsequent months.[21] Patients must use vigilant sun protection and hyperpigmentation can also be addressed with hydroquinones and low-potency topical steroids and the judicious use of retinoids.[4,10,22] Microdermabrasions and 20% to 30% salicylic acid peels may be helpful to the healing process.[17]

Hypopigmentation is caused by excessive heating, excessive cooling, or misaligned cooling.[23] It is permanent and may develop relative to background, untreated skin. Delayed hypopigmentation can also develop 6 to 12 months postoperatively in rare cases.[10] Patients who have a predisposition to develop hypopigmented scars or who have a significant level of sun damage before treatment may be at greater risk for delayed hypopigmentation. Patients who have had prior dermabrasion or deep peels are also at increased risk.[24]

Hypopigmentation can be minimized if entire cosmetic units or the whole face is resurfaced and the treatment is feathered into nearby areas, particularly the neck. As discussed previously, a medium-depth chemical peel may yield a uniform appearance to the face.[3] Excimer laser and topical photochemotherapy have also been shown to assist with repigmentation.[25]

Tattoo removal complications

Lasers may be used to remove or minimize tattoos by using the principles of selective photothermolysis, but tattoo removal carries a considerable color shift risk.[26] Laser treatment can deepen the colors of certain tattoos, and white, brown, and flesh-colored inks in particular can darken after laser treatment. Such color changes are thought caused by a redox reaction; it is thought that quality-switched laser treatment reduces some pigments, darkening rust-colored ferric to black ferrous oxide and white titanium^{4+} to blue titanium^{3+} dioxide.[27] An instance of tattoo brightening (brown lightening to orange and then lightening to yellow) has also been reported. Because dark tattoo inks are often a mix of several dark and light pigments, it is thought that in this case, the laser treatment selectively destroyed the darker chromophores, thus exposing the lighter chromophores and creating a brightening effect.[28] Currently, it is difficult to predict whether or not a color in a tattoo will shift. Tattoo artists often mix their own inks, and these pigment ingredients and tattoo age likely influence the skin's response to laser treatment. It is important to always test a small area of the tattoo first with the laser before beginning treatment.[27]

Color shift management depends on pigment ingredients, the anatomic location of the tattoo, the initial color of the tattoo, and whether or not the shift is temporary or permanent. Depending on the presentation, a treating physician may treat the tattoo with a different wavelength, select watchful waiting for an outcome, or consider alternate surgical options. If pigment fails to return to its original color after 4 months, it is considered a permanent shift.[26]

Recent developments in tattoo inks have sought to alleviate color shift problems altogether: Infinitink (Freedom2, Inc., Freedom Hill, New Jersey) is an ink that encapsulates tattoo pigments in microscopic beads coated with biodegradable plastic. The tattoos created with this ink are permanent until treated with a laser, which causes the beads to burst and release the tiny dye fragments into the bloodstream, thus standardizing the process of tattoo removal.[29]

Scarring

The risk of scarring due to laser treatment is small but noteworthy. Scars are more likely to develop after laser treatments involving a large number of passes, the use of excessive fluences, or improper pulse stacking (overlapping irradiated sites). Skin is especially vulnerable with ablative lasers. The risk of scarring can be minimized by the use of conservative parameters, judicious patient selection, scrupulous wound care post treatment, and sun avoidance. Prolonged erythema or eczematous changes can be early signs of scarring, and, as discussed previously, these warning signs should be addressed as soon as possible.[17] If hypertrophic or keloid scar tissue develops, it can be treated with topical and intralesional corticosteroids, silastic gel sheeting, or pressure dressings. A pulsed dye laser can also be used for the management of hypertrophic scars. Patients may also be referred to a laser surgeon for advanced management if appropriate.[10,17,30]

Infection

As with chemical peels, infections are of great concern during laser treatments and ablative laser resurfacing in particular, as the epidermis and portions of the dermis are removed. Physicians can greatly reduce the risk of postoperative infection by prophylactic administration of systemic antibiotics and proper postoperative topical treatments. Patients should always wash their hands thoroughly before touching their face and limit contact with small children and pets during recovery.[17]

Infections should be appropriately managed with the appropriate anti-infective treatment. Yeast infections, in particular candidiasis, are managed with systemic antifungals. Patients who are taking systemic antibiotics or who have a history of yeast infections should be evaluated on a case-by-case basis for antifungal prophylaxis.[8–10]

BOTULINUM TOXIN INJECTION COMPLICATIONS

Botulinum toxin type A received approval from the Food and Drug Administration for the treatment of strabismus and blepharospasm in 1989, cervical dystonia in 2000, and cosmetic use for glabellar wrinkles in 2002.[31] Currently, cosmetic botulinum toxin type A is marketed as Botox Cosmetic (Allergan) and Reloxin (Medicis Pharmaceutical).

The use of cosmetic botulinum toxin treatment is contraindicated in patients with certain pre-existing neuromuscular conditions, such as myasthenia gravis, and patients on certain medications (aminoglycosides, penicillamine, quinine, and calcium channel blockers).[32] Botulinum toxin is classified as pregnancy category C and thus should be avoided in pregnant or lactating women. There are no reports of complications in pregnant women, however, who experienced incidental exposure before learning of their pregnancy.[33]

The five primary facial targets indicated for botulinum toxin treatment are the frown lines of the glabella, the forehead, the periorbital rhytids (smile lines), the perioral lines (far more prominent in smokers), and the linear bands of the platysma. Treatment of the glabellar complex targets the procerus, corrugator supercilii, and depressor supercilii, and often includes the medial fibers of the orbicularis oculi and the frontalis, as these can intertwine with the corrugator (**Fig. 1**).[34,35] For treatment of the linear expression lines of the forehead, injections target the frontalis, the main muscle of the forehead and sole brow elevator. Periorbital injections target the lateral fibers of the orbicularis oculi. The orbicularis oculi is comprised of a palpebral section (covering the eyelid), the orbital section (surrounding the orbit from the lower forehead to upper cheek), and the lacrimal portion (the medial side of the orbit).[35] Perioral treatment targets the orbicularis oris, which, when injected with dermal fillers, can rejuvenate the aging lip; the depressor anguli oris, which helps revitalize a downturned mouth; and the mentalis to alleviate the appearance of a gummy smile (**Fig. 2**).[35] Injection of the platysmal bands can decrease the banding of the neck.

Common, Transient Complications

Common, short-term complications after botulinum toxin injections include pain, edema, ecchymosis, purpura, short-term hypesthesia, short-term headaches post injection, and, infrequently, prolonged migraines. The risks of dysesthesia and purpura may be minimized with the judicious use of pre-injection topical anesthetic and proper injection technique and the application of ice before and after the injection. Postinjection headaches are of two types: minor headaches, which may be treated with standard over-the-counter analgesics, and severe headaches, which are reported rarely and can be managed with stronger analgesics and oral corticosteroids when necessary.[36] Proper pretreatment counsel for patient avoidance of medications that hinder platelet function, such as nonsteroidal anti-inflammatory agents and aspirin, can lower the risk of purpura.[32,36] There are some anecdoctal data suggesting patients try using bromelain, found in pineapples; however, these reports are inconsistent.[37]

Significant Side Effects

Glabella complications

One of the most common complications of botulinum injections to the glabellar unit is a ptosis. It is thought caused by paralysis of the levator palpebrae muscle, potentially from the toxin's diffusion from another injection site.[31] For those patients affected, some improvement can be achieved with the use of α-adrenergic ophthalmic drops, which causes Müller's muscle to contract, elevating the lid (**Figs. 3** and **4**).[34]

Proper patient selection is crucial to reduce the risk of an upper lid ptosis. Upper lid ptosis may

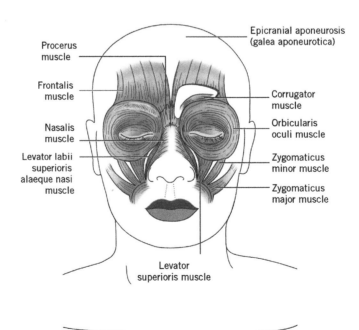

Fig. 1. Muscles of the upper and middle face. (*From* Hirsch R. Botulinum toxin. In: Sadick N, Lawrence N, Moy R, editors. Concise manual of cosmetic dermatologic surgery. New York: McGraw-Hill Medical; 2008. Fig. 5.1A; with permission.)

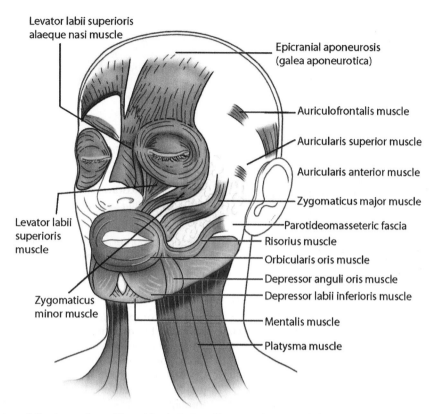

Levator labii superioris alaeque nasi muscle

Epicranial aponeurosis (galea aponeurotica)

Auriculofrontalis muscle

Auricularis superior muscle

Auricularis anterior muscle

Zygomaticus major muscle

Parotideomasseteric fascia

Risorius muscle

Orbicularis oris muscle

Depressor anguli oris muscle

Depressor labii inferioris muscle

Mentalis muscle

Platysma muscle

Levator labii superioris muscle

Zygomaticus minor muscle

Fig. 2. Muscles of the lower face. (*From* Hirsch R. Botulinum toxin. In: Sadick N, Lawrence N, Moy R, Hirsch RJ, editors. Concise manual of cosmetic dermatologic surgery. New York: McGraw-Hill Medical; 2008. Fig. 5.1B; with permission.)

result from the weakening of frontalis muscles that were being used to compensate for a pre-existing level of ptosis.[31] Pretreatment assessment of this ptosis is the best approach to prevent this unwanted effect.[34]

If lines on the side of the nose extending downwards (bunny lines) are treated in conjunction with the glabellar area, injections should avoid the levator labii alaeque nasi and the levator labii superioris to stop the upper lip from drooping (**Fig. 5**). Strong massage or downward massage may also result in lip ptosis.[35]

Forehead and brow complications

When treating the horizontal rhytids of the forehead, one way to assess the report from a patient of a "droop" is to ask the patient if it is easier or more difficult to apply eye makeup. It would be easier in the case of a lid ptosis and more difficult in the case of a brow ptosis. To avoid complications, injections to the frontalis should be placed 1 to 2 cm above the orbital rim to minimize diffusion (**Fig. 6**). Injecting a small amount of the toxin into the procerus may also prevent brow ptosis. Again, avoidance of simultaneous injection into

the brow depressors can avoid this risk and proper patient selection is critical.[35,38]

Injections to the medial portion of the frontalis without balanced injection of the lateral frontalis fibers can have untreated fibers pull the brow up. The resultant eyebrow is cock-eyed or looks surprised[32,38] (Spock's eyebrow) and is best corrected with the injection of a minute dose of botulinum toxin into the untreated lateral fibers (Ranella

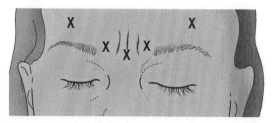

Fig. 3. Recommended injection sites for treating the muscles of the glabellar complex. (*From* Hirsch R. Botulinum toxin. In: Sadick N, Lawrence N, Moy R, Hirsch RJ, editors. Concise manual of cosmetic dermatologic surgery. New York: McGraw-Hill Medical; 2008. Figs. 5.2A and 5.2B; with permission.)

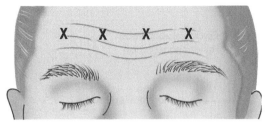

Fig. 4. Recommended injection sites for treating the muscles of the glabellar complex. (*From* Hirsch R. Botulinum toxin. In: Sadick N, Lawrence N, Moy R, Hirsch RJ, editors. Concise manual of cosmetic dermatologic surgery. New York: McGraw-Hill Medical; 2008. Figs. 5.2A and 5.2B; with permission.)

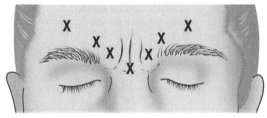

Fig. 6. Recommended injection sites for treatment of the frontalis. (*From* Hirsch R. Botulinum toxin. In: Sadick N, Lawrence N, Moy R, Hirsch RJ, editors. Concise manual of cosmetic dermatologic surgery. New York: McGraw-Hill Medical; 2008. Fig. 5.3A; with permission.)

Hirsch, MD personal communication with Alastair Carruthers, MD, October 2006).[38]

Periorbital complications

Any periorbital botulinum injection carries the risk of bruising, diplopia, ectropion, or a drooping orbicularis oculi. Should patients experience diplopia, covering or patching the eye alleviates some double vision.[32] To prevent diplopia, injections should be placed outside the bony orbital margin to prevent diffusion to the extraocular muscles.[39]

Cheek and lip ptosis may occur with inadvertent injection of the zygomaticus major muscle or the area below the zygomatic arch.[32,35,40] Injections to the orbicularis oculi to remedy crow's feet should be placed no lower than 1 cm above the zygomaticus notch to prevent possible midfacial and lip ptosis.[39]

These complications may be avoided by limiting the orbicularis oculi injection to approximately 1 cm outside the bony orbit or 1.5 cm lateral to the lateral canthus, carefully avoiding injection close to the inferior margin of the zygoma (**Fig. 7**). Clear visualization of the periocular musculature while injecting the toxin in a wheal or a series of continuous blebs with each injection occurring at the

advancing border of the preceding injection also lowers the risk of disruption.[32] Superficial injections are also known to minimize bruising.[35]

Perioral complications

Although the majority of injectable procedures of the lower face involve dermal fillers, the adjunctive use of botulinum toxin can be of value. To treat perioral lines, the orbicularis oris should be injected conservatively. This muscle can be injected through the upper and lower lip, and these injections should be symmetric and superficial (**Fig. 8**).[35,41]

Overtreatment of the orbicularis oris can cause significant side effects: patients may have problems pursing their lips, eating, or brushing their teeth. It may also lead to an asymmetric smile or speech impediments, including the inability to pronounce consonants, in particular "B" and "P," and decreased lip proprioception.[35] All patients must be warned of these potential complications, with special attention to those who earn a livelihood from their use (eg, professional musicians, newscasters, and actors).

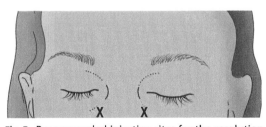

Fig. 5. Recommended injection sites for the resolution of bunny lines. The levator labii alaeque nasi and levator labii superioris should be avoided. (*From* Hirsch R. Botulinum toxin. In: Sadick N, Lawrence N, Moy R, Hirsch RJ, editors. Concise manual of cosmetic dermatologic surgery. New York: McGraw-Hill Medical; 2008. Fig. 5.5; with permission.)

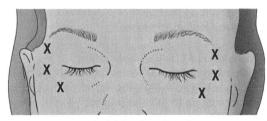

Fig. 7. Recommended injection sites for treatment of the periorbital musculature. It is important to avoid the zygomatus major and the area beneath the zygomatic arch. (*From* Hirsch R. Botulinum toxin. In: Sadick N, Lawrence N, Moy R, Hirsch RJ, editors. Concise manual of cosmetic dermatologic surgery. New York: McGraw-Hill Medical; 2008. Fig. 5.4A; with permission.)

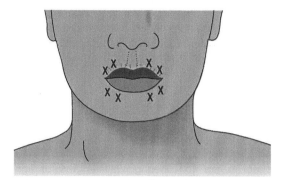

Fig. 8. Recommended injection sites for perioral musculature. Injections should be conservative, symmetric, and superficial within the muscles. (*From* Hirsch R. Botulinum toxin. In: Sadick N, Lawrence N, Moy R, Hirsch RJ, editors. Concise manual of cosmetic dermatologic surgery. New York: McGraw-Hill Medical; 2008. Fig. 5.6; with permission.)

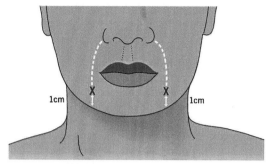

Fig. 9. Recommended injection sites for the treatment of the depressor anguli oris. Placement of the toxin is critical and should avoid the region closest to the mouth. (*From* Hirsch R. Botulinum toxin. In: Sadick N, Lawrence N, Moy R, Hirsch RJ, editors. Concise manual of cosmetic dermatologic surgery. New York: McGraw-Hill Medical; 2008. Fig. 5.7; with permission.)

Atrophy of the orbicularis oris may also cause the vermillion border to flatten secondarily. If flattening occurs, it can be corrected by injecting a dermal filler at the lip edge.[32] Injections placed too high above the orbicularis oris can lead the upper lip to invert, evert, or become temporarily ptotic.[35]

Contraction of the depressor anguli oris results in a frown, and the mouth can turn down at the edges permanently with age. This muscle can be treated with dermal fillers or botulinum toxin, which should be injected no higher than halfway between the lip and mandible to soften the labiomental fold (**Fig. 9**). The depressor anguli oris should be palpated to ensure correct placement.[38] If the depressor anguli oris is injected too close to the mouth, unilateral paralysis can result, which often can be distressing to patients.[35] An excellent technique is to first identify the muscle by instructing patients to clench their jaw. Botulinum toxin can then be injected into the inferior section of each depressor anguli oris muscle.[33]

Botulinum toxin injections to reduce the crease of nasolabial folds are rarely successful and are best avoided. Attempts to soften the nasolabial folds with botulinum toxin can lead to oral incompetence and difficulty with phonation.[31] In the majority of cases, patients respond better and report greater satisfaction using a dermal filler in this area.[32]

Mentalis and neck complications
Mentalis is usually injected with botulinum toxin lateral to midline on the chin to treat dimpling. Dimpling is caused by actions of the mentalis in addition to a loss of collagen and subcutaneous fat in the chin.[35,41] Inadvertent injection of the depressor labii can lead to lower lip depression. Some patients with dimpled chins may have hypertrophic mentalis muscles, a possible sign that patients may be especially vulnerable to oral incompetence, and these patients should not be injected in the mentalis.[35]

Overexuberant injections into the mental fold portion of mentalis may cause an incompetent mouth or asymmetric smile. Injecting into the mentalis at the point of the chin, however, may soften this area markedly. It is important to massage this region well after injection.[32]

Botulinum toxin may also be used for the treatment of platysmal bands and horizontal neck lines (**Fig. 10**). Patients with good skin elasticity and a minimal loss of submental fat may be good candidates for platysmal band injections.[35] The platysma is a superficial muscle and it is important

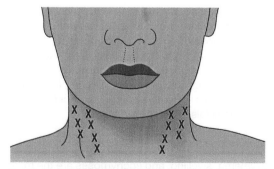

Fig. 10. Recommended injection sites for treatment of platysmal bands. The platysma is a superficial muscle and should be injected superficially to avoid adverse events. (*From* Hirsch R. Botulinum toxin. In: Sadick N, Lawrence N, Moy R, Hirsch RJ, editors. Concise manual of cosmetic dermatologic surgery. New York: McGraw-Hill Medical; 2008. Fig. 5.8; with permission.)

to avoid injecting too deeply, as this can yield potentially life-threatening dysphagia or voice changes.[38]

Systemic complications

Botulinum sensitization is a dose-dependent complication: cosmetic patients, who generally receive a maximum dose of 20 to 40 U, have a vastly lower risk of developing resistance than therapeutic botulinum patients, who can receive doses as high as 300 U. Among therapeutic patients, those who develop botulinum toxin resistence have been shown to have shorter dosing intervals, more booster doses, and higher treatment doses overall. It is also important to note that therapeutic patients can receive these higher doses as close as 8 weeks apart for many years.

Botulinum toxin resistance occurs when botulinum toxin–blocking antibodies form and prohibit any subsequent injections from having an effect. Antigenicity was a particular problem with older batches of the toxin, as these had a higher protein load (nanograms of botulinum toxin exposure per injection cycle). New batches have been reformulated with a lower protein content, reducing the probability of resistance. Although botulinum resistance is a concern for patients receiving therapeutic doses of the toxin, it is not a threat to cosmetic patients.[32,42–44]

Always the most serious and rare complication of botulinum toxin use is systemic botulism, but this is also not a significant threat to cosmetic patients. In the rare instances that cosmetic patients have contracted botulism, these cases involved unlicensed physicians administering research-grade botulinum toxin not licensed or intended for human use.[45,46]

DERMAL FILLER COMPLICATIONS

The multitude of available soft tissue fillers includes bovine and human collagens (Zyderm, Zyplast, CosmoDerm, and CosmoPlast), various members of the hyaluronan family (Restylane, Perlane, Juvederm, and Hylaform), calcium hydroxyapatite (Radiesse), poly-L-lactic acid (Sculptra), and synthetic polymers, such as liquid silicone and Artefill (also known as Artecoll).

Common, Transient Complications

Erythema, swelling, and ecchymoses are the most common and predictable side effects. Patients who drink alcohol or use blood thinners or certain herbal medications (vitamin E, feverfew, ginger, garlic, ginseng, and ginkgo) are at greater risk for purpura and should discontinue these substances at least 1 week before treatment (bleeding time

may take 2 to 3 weeks to correct fully).[47] Collagen-based products are less likely to produce local bruising than hyaluronic acid products, as the collagen products stimulate platelet activation.[48]

Significant Side Effects

Discoloration

Too superficial injections can cause blue-gray discoloration due to the Tyndall effect. The Tyndall effect refers to differing wavelengths of light scatter depending on the size of substances they encounter. According to Rayleigh scattering, for sufficiently small particles, the amount of light scattered is inversely proportional to the fourth power of the wavelength. For example, blue light is scattered more than red light by a factor of $(700/400)^4$, which equals approximately 10. Thus, within the skin, long red wavelengths can penetrate deeper into the tissue whereas shorter blue wavelengths are more easily scattered and reflected outwards.[49,50]

Placing a dermal filler at its intended depth is the key to preventing discoloration. Human collagen should be injected into the mid-dermis; medium-length hyaluronic acid fillers (Restylane and Juvederm) should be placed in the deep dermis[51]; calcium hydroxyapatite (Radiesse) should be injected at the dermal-subcutaneous border[52,53]; and fat and poly-L-lactic acid should be placed deeper in the subcutis.[54] There is a greater incidence of discoloration if a filler meant to be injected deep in the skin (eg, calcium hydroxyapatite) is placed within an area of limited dermis or subcutaneous tissue. These high-risk areas include the I-zone of the central face (the nasojugal folds, nasal dorsum, and lip); the infraorbital troughs; and fine superficial lines, such as periorbital and perioral rhytides (crow's feet and pucker lines).

Migration

Filler migration is usually reported with the nonbiodegradable fillers, and presentation may resemble a malignant neoplasm or granulomatous diseases.[55] Repositioning or removal of the nonbiodegradable implant may require wide tissue resections and complicated reconstructions.[56] Migration is not common with biodegradable fillers, although migration of longer-acting calcium hydroxyapatite has been reported regarding lip injections, which is why it is a contraindication by the manufacturer.[57]

Location corrections

The simplest, least expensive option for filler misplacement is manual extraction by gentle incising and removal. Douse-Dean and Jacob describe creating a small incision with a #11 blade in the area with the largest discoloration and applying gentle pressure with two opposing cotton swabs at either end of the discoloration stream. Rolling the swabs toward the incision, the filler should come out easily, and this can be repeated until all superficial filler is removed.[58]

Hyaluronidase injections are an effective aide for the management of the misplacement of hyaluronic acid and assist with the appearance of discoloration secondary to the Tyndall effect. This represents an off-label use of a product approved by the Food and Drug Administration. In 2007, Hirsch and Cohen[59] reported correcting a blue-gray infraorbital nasojugal nodule with hyaluronidase after treatment by an inexperienced injector.

In addition to use of hyaluronidase, the quality-switched 1064-nm laser can also be useful treatment for management of the Tyndall effect after dermal filler injections. Hirsch and colleagues reported two cases of successful treatment of Tyndall effect in the nasolabial folds.[60]

Allergic reaction and hypersensitivity

Bovine collagen injections (Zyderm and Zyplast) can rarely cause an allergic reaction. Signs of hypersensitivity include erythema, edema induration, pruritus, and pain. Best practice is double skin allergy testing performed 2 weeks apart,[55] conducted with commercially available Zyderm test syringes. Contraindications to testing and treatment include allergy to lidocaine or bovine collagen.[61]

Hyaluronic acid fillers generally do not require skin testing.[62] Hyaluronidase injections can help with hypersensitivity reactions with hyaluronic acid products should they occur.[63] Adverse reactions when reported are most frequently local injection-site reactions.[64]

Granulomas

Foreign body granulomas are aggregates of particular types of chronic inflammatory cells that create nodules a few millimeters in diameter. Histologically, they are characterized by histiocytes, epithelioid histiocytes, and multinucleated giant cells contained by lymphocytes and containing amorphous material.[65] Granulomas from hyaluronic acid fillers may be caused by an allergy to the material or an immunologic response to the protein contaminants in the hyaluronic acid preparations; these reactions can be treated with hyaluronidase.[66,67]

Granulomas are most common in patients injected with nonbiodegradable or slowly biodegradable fillers.[55] They may appear within 6 to 15 months post injection. Intralesional steroids or prednisone in dosages of up to 60 mg per day may be used to treat granulomas, although atrophy may occur with overzealous therapy.[66,67] Lemperle and colleagues[68] suggest surgical excision as a last resort generally reserved for granulomas on the lips or those in the subcutaneous fat.

Infection

Infection is a rare and early complication after injection with fillers. Lesions of early infection occur up to several days post treatment and are difficult to identify, given their similarities to an inflammatory response. Early lesions may resolve spontaneously or require minimal medical interference.

Late infection is usually caused by common skin and soft tissue pathogens, including *Streptococcus aureus*.[55] Late infection is defined as appearing 8 to 12 days after injection and can be described as granulomatous tissue reactions, granulomatous allergic tissue reactions developing into abscesses, or nodules.[69] For temporary fillers, the infection may disappear spontaneously as the filler degrades. Infections caused by longer-lasting fillers may be treated with high doses of a broad-spectrum antibiotic for 7 days.[8,69]

Lesions that develop more than 2 weeks post procedure suggest the presence of an atypical infection, and mycobacteria is a frequent culprit.[55] A firm, slightly tender mass or nodule with or without fluid may appear. Systemic reactions, including fever, leukocytosis, weight loss, and fatigue, may also occur. Lesions should be aspirated or biopsied, and up to four antimicrobial agents may be used if the infection is mycobacterial. Disrupting or removing the lesion may also speed recovery.[55]

Infection may also be due to tainted product, as in the case of a 2002 outbreak of *Mycobacterium abscessus* infections. In this case, nonphysicians were injecting a tainted, gray market hyaluronic acid derivative.[70] Such impurities were attributed to faults in the manufacturing process.[70]

Necrosis

Injection necrosis is a rare but serious potential complication caused by compromise of the vascular supply to the treated area by compression, injury, or obstruction of the vessels.[71,72] Necrosis has occurred with every type of filler.[48] It is of particular risk in the glabellar area, where blockage of the central artery under the glabellar area can lead to embolism to the ophthalmic artery and vision loss. Perioral injections are also of risk because of the circumoral artery.[48] Warning signs of occlusion preceding necrosis include imme-diate severe pain and blanching of the skin.[48]

If obstruction is suspected, immediately cease the injecting, and vigorous massage may break up the clot or filler. In this case, postmassage hyperemia can be an important sign of resolu-tion.[48] Given their thickness, collagen filler deposits are more difficult to disrupt with massage than hyaluronic acid products. Warm compresses should be applied to promote local vasodilation, and topical 2% nitroglycerin paste may be applied if necessary, as this encourages pharmacologic vasodilation. As with massage, collagen-induced occlusions are less responsive to these remedies than hyaluronic acid fillers.[48] In 2007, Hirsch and colleagues[73] described the first known hyaluronic acid embolic event successfully managed with hyaluronidase, and subsequent cases of success-ful management with hyaluronidase have been reported.[74]

Rigorous attention to detail and advanced injec-tion technique can greatly reduce the risk of necrosis, but obstructions may be unavoidable in some patients. It is recommended that physicians use 30-gauge or smaller needles when injecting risky sites, as the pressure when injecting provides helpful feedback to the injector.[48] Close attention to the cutaneous surface is also critical.

SUMMARY

Although today's cosmetic rejuvenation options are not risk-free, serious complications are rare. Chemical peels, laser treatments, botulinum toxin, and dermal fillers all offer significant nonsurgical rejuvenation options for the aging face. Although it is important for patients to consider benefits versus risks whenever choosing a cosmetic proce-dure, patients seeking rejuvenation today have a range of low-risk options that offer significant aesthetic improvement without the risks or costs of surgery.

REFERENCES

1. Klein AW. Complications and adverse reactions with the use of botulinum toxin. Dis Mon 2002;48:336–56.
2. Cassano N, Alessandrini G, Mastrolonardo M, et al. Peeling agents: toxicological and allergological aspects. J Eur Acad Dermatol Venereol 1999;13: 14–23.
3. Monheit GD. Chemical peels. Skin Therapy Lett 2004;9:6–11.
4. Coleman WP 3rd. Dermal peels. Dermatol Clin 2001; 19:405–11.
5. Brody HJ. Complications of chemical resurfacing. Dermatol Clin 2001;19:427–38, vii–viii.
6. Rubin MG. Complications. In: Manual of chemical peels: superficial and medium depth. 1st edition. New York: Lippincott Williams and Wilkins; 1995. p. 130–54.
7. Kovach BT, Sengelmann RD. Chemical peels. In: Hirsch RJ, Cohen JL, Sadick N, editors. Regional approach to aethetic rejuvenation. New York: McGraw-Hill Medical; 2009. p. 81–8.
8. Strauss RA. Management of infections associated with laser-assisted cosmetic skin resurfacing. Oral Maxillofac Surg Clin North Am 2003;15:147–53.
9. Manuskiatti W, Fitzpatrick RE, Goldman MP, et al. Prophylactic antibiotics in patients undergoing laser resurfacing of the skin. J Am Acad Dermatol 1999; 40:77–84.
10. Alexiades-Armenakas MR, Dover JS, Arndt KA. The spectrum of laser skin resurfacing: nonablative, frac-tional, and ablative laser resurfacing. J Am Acad Dermatol 2008;58:719–37 [quiz 738–40].
11. Alster T, Zaulyanov L. Laser scar revision: a review. Dermatol Surg 2007;33:131–40.
12. Alster TS. Laser treatment of hypertrophic scars, keloids, and striae. Dermatol Clin 1997;15:419–29.
13. Niessen FB, Spauwen PH, Schalkwijk J, et al. On the nature of hypertrophic scars and keloids: a review. Plast Reconstr Surg 1999;104:1435–58.
14. Marneros AG, Norris JE, Watanabe S, et al. Genome scans provide evidence for keloid susceptibility loci on chromosomes 2q23 and 7p11. J Invest Dermatol 2004;122:1126–32.
15. Marneros AG, Norris JE, Olsen BR, et al. Clinical genetics of familial keloids. Arch Dermatol 2001; 137:1429–34.
16. Lapidoth M, Yagima Odo ME, Odo LM. Novel use of erbium:YAG (2,940-nm) laser for fractional ablative photothermolysis in the treatment of photodamaged facial skin: a pilot study. Dermatol Surg 2008;34: 1048–53.
17. Willey A, Anderson RR, Azpiazu JL, et al. Complica-tions of laser dermatologic surgery. Lasers Surg Med 2006;38:1–15.
18. Narins RS, Tope WD, Pope K, et al. Overtreatment effects associated with a radiofrequency tissue-tightening device: rare, preventable, and correctable with subcision and autologous fat trans-fer. Dermatol Surg 2006;32:115–24.
19. Graber EM, Tanzi EL, Alster TS. Side effects and complications of fractional laser photothermolysis: experience with 961 treatments. Dermatol Surg 2008;34:301–5 [discussion 305–7].
20. Ward PD, Baker SR. Long-term results of carbon dioxide laser resurfacing of the face. Arch Facial Plast Surg 2008;10:238–43 [discussion 244–5].
21. Goldberg DJ. Nonablative laser surgery for pig-mented skin. Dermatol Surg 2005;31:1263–7.
22. Bernstein LJ, Kauvar AN, Grossman MC, et al. The short- and long-term side effects of carbon

dioxide laser resurfacing. Dermatol Surg 1997;23: 519–25.

23. Hirsch RJ, Anderson RR. Principles of laser-skin interactions. senior editors. Horn TD, Mascaro JM, Saurat JH, Mancini AJ, Salasche SJ, Stingl G. In: Bolognia JL, Jorizzo JL, Rapini RP, editors. Dermatology. London: Mosby; 2003. p. 2143–51.

24. Goldberg DJ. Complications in laser resurfacing. In: Complications in cutaneous laser surgery. 1st edition. New York: Taylor and Francis; 2004. p. 27–71.

25. Bhatt N, Alster TS. Laser surgery in dark skin. Dermatol Surg 2008;34:184–94 [discussion 194–5].

26. Peach AH, Thomas K, Kenealy J. Colour shift following tattoo removal with Q-switched Nd-YAG laser (1064/532). Br J Plast Surg 1999;52:482–7.

27. Holzer AM, Burgin S, Levine VJ. Adverse effects of Q-switched laser treatment of tattoos. Dermatol Surg 2008;34:118–22.

28. Jimenez G, Weiss E, Spencer JM. Multiple color changes following laser therapy of cosmetic tattoos. Dermatol Surg 2002;28:177–9.

29. Conroy E. New tattoo ink erases any regrets. content via Associated Press. Available at: http://www.usatoday.com/tech/science/discoveries/2007-07-19-tatoo-combustible-ink_N.htm. Accessed December 07, 2008.

30. Stier MF, Hirsch RJ. Rejuvenation of scars and striae. In: Hirsch RJ, Cohen JL, Sadick N, editors. Aesthetic rejuvenation: a regional approach. New York: McGraw-Hill Medical; 2009. p. 210–34.

31. Spiegel JH. Treatment of periorbital rhytids with botulinum toxin type A: maximizing safety and results. Arch Facial Plast Surg 2005;7:198–202.

32. Klein AW. Complications, adverse reactions, and insights with the use of botulinum toxin. Dermatol Surg 2003;29:549–56 [discussion 556].

33. Neuhaus IM, Yu SS. Botulinum toxin. In: Hirsch RJ, Cohen JL, Sadick N, editors. Aesthetic rejuvenation: a regional approach. New York: McGraw-Hill Medical; 2009. p. 64–71.

34. Balikian RV, Zimbler MS. Primary and adjunctive uses of botulinum toxin type A in the periorbital region. Otolaryngol Clin North Am 2007;40:291–303.

35. Carruthers J, Fagien S, Matarasso SL. Consensus recommendations on the use of botulinum toxin type a in facial aesthetics. Plast Reconstr Surg 2004;114:1S–22S.

36. Alam M, Arndt KA, Dover JS. Severe, intractable headache after injection with botulinum a exotoxin: report of 5 cases. J Am Acad Dermatol 2002;46: 62–5.

37. Baumann L. Botanical ingredients in cosmeceuticals. J Drugs Dermatol 2007;6:1084–8.

38. Carruthers JD, Glogau RG, Blitzer A. Advances in facial rejuvenation: botulinum toxin type a, hyaluronic acid dermal fillers, and combination therapies—consensus recommendations. Plast Reconstr Surg 2008;121:5S–30S.

39. Hirsch RJ. Botulinum toxin. In: Sadick N, Lawrence N, Moy R, Hirsch RJ, editors. Concise manual of cosmetic dermatologic surgery. New York: McGraw-Hill Medical; 2008. p. 47–56.

40. Fedok FG. Advances in minimally invasive facial rejuvenation. Curr Opin Otolaryngol Head Neck Surg 2008;16:359–68.

41. Suryadevara AC. Update on perioral cosmetic enhancement. Curr Opin Otolaryngol Head Neck Surg 2008;16:347–51.

42. Borodic G, Johnson E, Goodnough M, et al. Botulinum toxin therapy, immunologic resistance, and problems with available materials. Neurology 1996; 46:26–9.

43. Mahajan ST, Brubaker L. Botulinum toxin: from life-threatening disease to novel medical therapy. Am J Obstet Gynecol 2007;196:7–15.

44. Greene P, Fahn S, Diamond B. Development of resistance to botulinum toxin type A in patients with torticollis. Mov Disord 1994;9:213–7.

45. Chertow DS, Tan ET, Maslanka SE, et al. Botulism in 4 adults following cosmetic injections with an unlicensed, highly concentrated botulinum preparation. JAMA 2006;296:2476–9.

46. Souayah N, Karim H, Kamin SS, et al. Severe botulism after focal injection of botulinum toxin. Neurology 2006;67:1855–6.

47. Ciocon JO, Ciocon DG, Galindo DJ. Dietary supplements in primary care. Botanicals can affect surgical outcomes and follow-up. Geriatrics 2004;59:20–4.

48. Narins RS, Jewell M, Rubin M, et al. Clinical conference: management of rare events following dermal fillers—focal necrosis and angry red bumps. Dermatol Surg 2006;32:426–34.

49. Suhai B, Horvath G. How well does the Rayleigh model describe the E-vector distribution of skylight in clear and cloudy conditions? A full-sky polarimetric study. J Opt Soc Am A Opt Image Sci Vis 2004;21:1669–76.

50. Anderson RR. Rest azured? J Am Acad Dermatol 2001;44:874–5.

51. Narins RS, Brandt F, Leyden J, et al. A randomized, double- blind, multicenter comparison of the efficacy and tolerability of Restylane versus Zyplast for the correction of nasolabial folds. Dermatol Surg 2003;29:588–95.

52. Berlin A, Cohen JL, Goldberg DJ. Calcium hydroxylapatite for facial rejuvenation. Semin Cutan Med Surg 2006;25:132–7.

53. Roy D, Sadick N, Mangat D. Clinical trial of a novel filler material for soft tissue augmentation of the face containing synthetic calcium hydroxylapatite microspheres. Dermatol Surg 2006;32: 1134–9.

54. Vleggaar D. Soft-tissue augmentation and the role of poly-L-lactic acid. Plast Reconstr Surg 2006;118: 46S–54S.

55. Lowe NJ, Maxwell CA, Patnaik R. Adverse reactions to dermal fillers: review. Dermatol Surg 2005;31: 1616–25.

56. Rzany B, Zielke H. Complications. In: de Maio M, Rzany B, editors. Injectable fillers in aesthetic medicine. 1st edition. New York: Springer; 2006. p. 67–77.

57. Beer KR. Radiesse nodule of the lips from a distant injection site: report of a case and consideration of etiology and management. J Drugs Dermatol 2007; 6:846–7.

58. Douse-Dean T, Jacob CI. Fast and easy treatment for reduction of the Tyndall effect secondary to cosmetic use of hyaluronic acid. J Drugs Dermatol 2008;7:281–3.

59. Hirsch RJ, Cohen JL. Challenge: correcting superficially placed hyaluronic acid. Skin Aging 2007;15: 36–8.

60. Hirsch RJ, Narurkar V, Carruthers J. Management of injected hyaluronic acid induced Tyndall effects. Lasers Surg Med 2006;38:202–4.

61. Cheng JT, Perkins SW, Hamilton MM. Collagen and injectable fillers. Otolaryngol Clin North Am 2002; 35:73–85, vi.

62. Friedman PM, Mafong EA, Kauvar AN, et al. Safety data of injectable nonanimal stabilized hyaluronic acid gel for soft tissue augmentation. Dermatol Surg 2002;28:491–4.

63. Lupo MP. Hyaluronic acid fillers in facial rejuvenation. Semin Cutan Med Surg 2006;25:122–6.

64. Nathan N, Benrhaiem M, Lotfi H, et al. The role of hyaluronidase on lidocaine and bupivacaine pharmacokinetics after peribulbar blockade. Anesth Analg 1996;82:1060–4.

65. Salmi R, Boari B, Manfredini R. Siliconoma: an unusual entity for the internist. Am J Med 2004;116:67.

66. Brody HJ. Use of hyaluronidase in the treatment of granulomatous hyaluronic acid reactions or unwanted hyaluronic acid misplacement. Dermatol Surg 2005;31:893–7.

67. Lowe NJ, Maxwell CA, Lowe P, et al. Hyaluronic acid skin fillers: adverse reactions and skin testing. J Am Acad Dermatol 2001;45:930–3.

68. Lemperle G, Rullan PP, Gauthier-Hazan N. Avoiding and treating dermal filler complications. Plast Reconstr Surg 2006;118:92S–107S.

69. Christensen L. Normal and pathologic tissue reactions to soft tissue gel fillers. Dermatol Surg 2007; 33(Suppl 2):S168–75.

70. Toy BR, Frank PJ. Outbreak of Mycobacterium abscessus infection after soft tissue augmentation. Dermatol Surg 2003;29:971–3.

71. Coleman SR. Avoidance of arterial occlusion from injectable fillers. Aesthetic Surg J 2002;22:555.

72. Schanz S, Schippert W, Ulmer A, et al. Arterial embolization caused by injection of hyaluronic acid (Restylane). Br J Dermatol 2002;146:928–9.

73. Hirsch RJ, Cohen JL, Carruthers JD. Successful management of an unusual presentation of impending necrosis following a hyaluronic acid injection embolus and a proposed algorithm for management with hyaluronidase. Dermatol Surg 2007;33:357–60.

74. Hirsch RJ, Lupo M, Cohen JL, et al. Delayed presentation of impending necrosis following soft tissue augmentation with hyaluronic acid and successful management with hyaluronidase. J Drugs Dermatol 2007;6:325–8.

Emerging Technologies in Aesthetic Medicine

Bobby Y. Reddy, MSa, Basil M. Hantash, MD, PhDb,*

KEYWORDS

- Laser technologies • Skin rejuvenation • Ultrasound
- Microdermabrasion • Acne vulgaris • Lipolysis and cellulite

The advent of novel technologies for aesthetic indications has transformed the delivery of skin care in clinical dermatology. The harmful effects of UV irradiation have led to the development of a wide array of treatments aimed at reversing photodamage. One rapidly growing area of skin rejuvenation therapies is laser technology. Ablative lasers (CO_2 and erbium:YAG) have demonstrated unparalleled effectiveness in their ability to treat sun-induced skin damage. Hence, these devices remain the gold standard for skin rejuvenation. However, ablative lasers are associated with significant side effects including delayed erythema and edema, pigmentation abnormalities, significant scarring and increased risk of infection.[1–4] Furthermore, their use also requires a lengthened downtime or period of time after the procedure that patients cannot perform routine activities.[5] These troublesome complications have limited the use of ablative laser devices in clinical practice. Since then, nonablative and fractional lasers have become popular therapeutic options without the side effects associated with ablative procedures. More recently, in light of the efficacy observed with ablative lasers and the success of fractional devices, ablative fractional systems have been introduced, merging the two modalities to deliver exceptional results.[6] This article discusses novel research and emerging technologies in skin rejuvenation. In addition, recent technological interventions for acne vulgaris, lipolysis, and cellulite are also addressed.

AN OVERVIEW OF LASERS AND SKIN REJUVENATION

Rhytides (wrinkles) and skin laxity constitute the primary aesthetically undesired effects of photodamage. All laser and light-based therapies aim to reduce wrinkles without compromising the integrity of the deeper tissue layers. Ablative devices completely eliminate the epidermis and the upper layers of the dermis, inducing the formation of a wound.[6] This lesion subsequently reconstitutes an epithelium in approximately 7 to 14 days.[6,7] In addition to the generation of a wound, ablative therapies also have an important effect on collagen coagulation through the delivery of thermal energy to the surrounding connective tissue.[6] Nonablative lasers heat the deep dermal layers while simultaneously cooling the epidermis.[8] This process achieves the desired effect of dermal regeneration without damaging the epidermal barrier. Although greatly diminishing the adverse effects associated with ablative therapies, a significant loss in clinical efficacy is encountered using nonablative systems.[9] These challenges have led to the emergence of fractional lasers. Fractional devices produce distinct lesions of thermal damage surrounded by larger zones of undisturbed normal skin.[10] The combination of lesions and adjacent viable tissue allows for complete reepithelization within 24 to 48 hours and creates an annular coagulation of collagen, which serves to tighten skin.[11] Fractional lasers are also associated with minimal posttreatment

a Department of Dermatology, New Jersey Medical School, Newark, NJ, USA
b Department of Surgery, Division of Plastic Surgery, Stanford University School of Medicine, 257 Campus Drive, Stanford, CA 94305-5148, USA
* Corresponding author.
E-mail address: basil@elixirinstitute.org (B.M. Hantash).

Dermatol Clin 27 (2009) 521–527
doi:10.1016/j.det.2009.08.004
0733-8635/09/$ – see front matter © 2009 Published by Elsevier Inc.

care and lack the significant side effects associated with ablative therapies.

Through different mechanisms, all laser therapies utilize thermal energy to reform and homogenize connective tissue. Initially, there is a localized coagulation of collagen fibers for 14 days post-treatment, and this process is followed by new connective tissue synthesis from the thermally altered matrix.[6,7] Histologically, fibroblasts may be observed migrating to the affected regions and initiating new collagen formation.[12] The entire process is mediated through the activation of various cytokines and molecular pathways, and culminates in increased elasticity and improved aesthetic appearance of skin.[13]

EMERGING THERAPIES
Fractional Lasers

The emergence of fractional resurfacing or fractional photothermolysis (FP) has significantly advanced laser skin therapy. The first fractional device approved for clinical use was the non-ablative laser Fraxel (Reliant Technologies, Mountain View, California).[10] This 1550 nm erbium-doped fiber laser was designed to generate microscopic treatment zones (MTZ), areas of thermal necrosis surrounded by viable tissue.[7] This mixture, resulting from interlesional sparing, allows for rapid reepithelialization of thermally damaged zones.[14] Fraxel maintains an undamaged stratum corneum, which greatly reduces the risk of developing a bacterial infection resulting from treatment.[10] Furthermore, the preserved epidermal barrier serves to function in exfoliating underlying coagulated tissue, referred to as microepidermal necrotic debris (MEND).[10] Studies have demonstrated that MEND contains melanin and elastin.[10] The transepidermal elimination of melanin may explain the observed efficacy of FP in the treatment of melasma.[15] Complete regeneration using this device takes approximately 3 months, and it involves the recruitment of various cytokines and mediators, such as heat shock proteins and transforming growth factor-β (TGF-β).[10] An important technical feature of the Fraxel laser is the Intelligent Optical Tracking system (IOTS), which serves to remove the necessity of stationary treatment. The IOTS allows for the production of constant density MTZ while screening the physician's hand speed, preventing nonuniform treatment distributions.[10] Prior to the emergence of IOTS and FP, treatment for skin rejuvenation was restricted to the face because of the risks of scarring and hyperpigmentation associated with treating other areas. The Fraxel laser coagulates approximately 20% of the target zone, hence the risk of collateral thermal damage is drastically diminished.[10] This

advantage has allowed for efficacious treatment of nonfacial areas with short healing periods.[16] Because of rapid healing and few side effects, this device proved to be a more convenient and safer treatment option than the existing ablative and nonablative lasers. The potential therapeutic benefits of this revolutionary device are only beginning to unravel.

Since then, other fractional laser therapies have emerged, steadily enhancing the options for treatment. The 1540 nm-pulsed device, Lux 1540 Fractional (Palomar Medical Technologies, Burlington, Massachusetts), has been approved by the US Food and Drug Administration for soft-tissue coagulation.[17,18] This device includes a convenient handpiece connected to a pulsed light and laser system that delivers microbeams of pulsed light capable of penetrating 1mm of skin.[17] A major benefit of this system is the fact that it is completely painless, making it a reliable option for patients who are especially intolerant to pain.[17] Another new fractional system is the Affirm laser (Cynosure Inc., Westford, Massachusetts), which sequentially emits two different laser wavelengths (1320 nm and 1440 nm).[17] This device utilizes a unique microlens array to dispense laser light at two wavelengths through a network of microbeams, allowing for high-intensity penetration of the superficial and deep layers of skin.[17] Unlike the Fraxel laser, this system does not require a tracking dye and is associated with much less pain, as a result of the more superficial microtreatment zones.[19]

Recently, fractional ablative lasers based on CO_2 and heated Er:YAG systems have also been introduced. The 10,600 nm AFR system (Reliant Technologies Inc.) is the prototype fractional ablative CO_2 laser.[20] This novel device generates MTZ with variable depths and widths through manipulation of pulse energy delivery.[21] These areas of tissue ablation are bordered by zones of tissue coagulation, representing denatured collagen.[22] There is an annular ring pattern of coagulation surrounding the microlesions generated with AFR treatment.[20] This annular configuration of thermal coagulation may serve to enhance tissue tightening benefits because of collagen shortening in a three-dimensional mechanism.[21] Treatment with this device also employs transepidermal exfoliation of MEND, as observed with nonablative fractional photothermolysis. Furthermore, immunohistochemical studies of treated skin demonstrated the induction of epidermal heat shock proteins and a significant collagen remodeling/wound healing response lasting 3 months.[21]

Fractional ablative resurfacing may also be performed through Er:YAG lasers. The prototype 2940 nm Er:YAG laser Pixel (Alma Lasers Ltd,

Caesarea, Israel) has also demonstrated promising results in the treatment of photodamaged skin.[23] This device delivers laser microbeams through a matrixed microlens to create highly precise ablation zones, referred to as pixels.[23] Collateral damage may be restricted by regulating the number of laser passes, matrix size, and level of energy applied.[23] In a pilot study, all subjects treated with this device for skin rejuvenation experienced favorable results that lasted at least 2 months posttreatment, and an evaluation at 6 to 9 months after treatment revealed that a majority maintained their results.[23] Furthermore, this study was devoid of any significant adverse effects, including hyperpigmentation, a particularly distressing side effect of ablative lasers.[23] Therefore, fractional ablative lasers may serve as a trustworthy option for skin rejuvenation, minimizing the risks associated with conventional ablative lasers while exhibiting an increased efficacy compared with nonablative devices.[20,22]

Radiofrequency

In recent years, radiofrequency (RF) systems have generated growing interest because of their effectiveness in reducing rhytides and skin laxity. RF devices generate electrical energy that heats the dermis at comparatively low temperatures.[17] The prototype system was the monopolar RF device ThermaCool (Thermage, Inc., Hayward, California).[24,25] This device was designed to uniformly heat the reticular dermis utilizing the tissue's inherent resistance to current flow.[17] The electric field of polarity is varied at a frequency of 6 million times per second, inducing charged particles in the electric field to change orientation at that speed, and as a result, heat derives from the tissue's resistance to the rapid displacement of particles.[17] This device was received with marked enthusiasm for its potential to produce skin tightening with minimal downtime. In addition, side effects were limited to minimal postoperative erythema, which disappeared within hours.[17] However, the results of the system were inconsistent and often statistically insignificant after photographic analysis.[26] These shortcomings lead to development of combinatory therapy, using electrical and optical energies. The combination of modalities was found to enhance the skin rejuvenation accomplished by either treatment alone.[27-29] The synergistic effect of infrared laser at 900 nm with bipolar RF and intense pulsed light (500–1200 nm) has demonstrated significant reduction of all types of photodamage and rhytides.[17] However, a major drawback of this therapy is the necessity of numerous treatments at 2- to 3-week intervals,

which may ultimately result in only 25% improvement.[30] Hence, the extensive costs and procedural times in combination with marginal benefits served to limit the clinical use of this approach.

Newer RF technologies have emerged with more promising potential since then. The latest of which is the novel fractional RF device, Renesis (Primaeva Medical, Inc., Fremont, California).[1] This system foregoes the noninvasive modes of predecessor RF devices with the development of a minimally invasive bipolar microneedle delivery system.[1] Renesis generates localized coagulation zones within the reticular dermis characterized as radiofrequency thermal zones.[1] This fractional radiofrequency system offers controlled dermal heating through pulse duration variance, allowing for fractional sparing of the epidermis and important adnexal structures.[1] An interesting feature of this device is the Intelligent Feedback System (IFS), a temperature sensor that offers real-time feedback of skin temperature from within the developing lesion.[1] Before delivering RF energy, IFS also performs a test current that generates information pertaining to tissue impedance and location of electrodes.[1] These details allow for the apparatus to calculate the optimal heat delivery for each unique target tissue.[1] This state-of-the-art technology facilitates the creation of precise thermal zones with minimal collateral damage. Furthermore, Renesis is associated with a remarkable wound-healing response by way of the recruitment heat shock proteins and inflammatory mediators, such as TNF-α, IL-β, and TGF-β.[31] In a prospective clinical study, histologic analysis of subjects revealed new collagen deposition at 10 weeks posttreatment, characterized by increased cellularity and hyaluronic deposits.[31] In addition, histologic studies also demonstrated increased elastin content in the same time interval.[31] In summary, the remarkable efficacy in microdermal ablation, combined with the evidence of marked neocollagenesis and neoelastogenesis, suggests that Renesis may become a dependable treatment choice for rhytids and skin laxity.

Ultrasound

Ultrasound therapy, which in the past has been a treatment option for diminishing solid tumors, is now being explored as a modality for skin rejuvenation.[32] Ultrasound treatment delivers heat to the dermis through the absorption of acoustic energy.[33] The cellular response to the thermal damage is dependent on the temperature utilized, exposure time, and the recruitment of specific cytokines and inflammatory mediators.[34] Hence, the mechanism of dermal remodeling shares many similarities with changes induced by laser- and light-based devices. The classic high-intensity focused ultrasound (HIFU) application has been proven effective as a noninvasive means to induce thermal damage.[35] This approach delivers high-powered acoustic energy with the aim of debulking target tissue.[32] However, a drawback of HIFU therapy is the limitation to macroscopic applications, which makes it impractical for skin rejuvenation.[32] As a result, intense focused ultrasound (IFUS) has been developed with the aim of inducing precise microcoagulation within the skin.[32] The prototype IFUS device Ulthera (Ulthera Inc., Mesa, Arizona) presents as a novel therapeutic option for skin rejuvenation.[32] In contrast to HIFU, this device delivers significantly shorter pulses of energy in the millisecond range (50–200ms).[32] Furthermore, this device operates at a frequency in the megahertz range, compared to the kilohertz range used by HIFU.[32] These modifications, combined with sharp focusing, allow this system to effectively generate microscopic thermal damage while delivering significantly lower energy than HIFU.[32] The IFUS approach is able to create well-defined areas of thermal coagulation within the reticular dermis without disrupting the epidermis and papillary dermis.[32] Furthermore, simultaneous cooling is not required to maintain the epidermis with this modality. Another major advantage of Ulthera for skin rejuvenation is the fact that ultrasound energy is independent of chromophores for energy absorption.[36] Acoustic energy generated by ultrasound is absorbed by the mechanical composition of target tissue.[32] In contrast, many conventional laser- and light-based therapies require melanin as a chromophore, which makes treatment for darker skin types problematic.[32] Ulthera circumvents this common dilemma and serves as a suitable therapy for patients who have darker skin. These promising features indicate that IFUS may soon become one of the leading options for noninvasive skin treatments.

Microdermabrasion

Microdermabrasion is an exceedingly popular procedure for superficial skin resurfacing. This technique was first introduced in Italy in 1985, and it has recently become one of the most desired aesthetic treatments internationally.[37] The American Society of Plastic Surgeons reported that 1,032,417 microdermabrasion procedures were performed in the United States in 2002 alone.[37] Although this technique has been extremely prevalent for many years, the biological

mechanisms underlying its efficacy are only recently beginning to be uncovered. The procedure involves the deposition of microcrystals, usually aluminum oxide (sodium chloride, magnesium oxide, and sodium bicarbonate are other options), on the surface of the skin with rapid strokes of a handpiece.[38] Meanwhile, an aspiration tube attached to the handpiece vacuums the crystals and skin debris. The skin depth of the procedure is established by the strength of crystal flow, speed of handpiece movement, and the number of passes on the target region.[37] The procedure ultimately induces the emergence of newer skin cells underlying the stratum corneum to surface, which serves to enhance the aesthetic appearance of the treatment zone. In addition to treating photodamage, this procedure has been widely used as therapy for acne scarring and post-inflammatory hyperpigmentation.[39] Recently, research has aimed to explore the molecular changes resulting from microdermabrasion.[40] Previously, it was suggested that microdermabrasion stimulated the emergence of new cells through the removal and disruption of the stratum corneum.[37,39] However, this theory has been challenged by recent histologic evidence that shows a completely intact stratum corneum following microdermabrasion treatment.[40] A new hypothesis states that microdermabrasion may stimulate skin regeneration by inducing molecular changes within the dermis through mechanical stretch effects on the stratum corneum, rather than removal or disruption.[40] Recent studies have reported that microdermabrasion treatment triggers a cascade of molecular events which induce marked dermal collagen remodeling and repair.[41] This process involves the activation of the cytokines AP-1, NF-κB, TNF-α and IL-1β, which collectively serve to upregulate the expression of various connective tissue degrading enzymes.[41] This molecular cascade shares similarities with the remodeling mechanisms demonstrated to be significant in the repair of photodamage and wound healing induced by carbon dioxide laser resurfacing.[41] These novel insights set the path for the development of more efficacious technology for microdermabrasion applications.

Acne Vulgaris Treatment

Acne vulgaris is a prevalent skin disease involving the pilosebaceous unit. Studies have reported that the aesthetic concerns relating to acne may have an effect on patients' psychological health equivalent to that of chronic systemic conditions, such as diabetes, arthritis, and epilepsy.[42] Therefore, efficacious therapy will serve to profoundly impact the quality of life of patients who have this disease. Currently, topical and oral medications, including retinoids, benzoyl peroxide, and antibiotics, comprise the core treatment regimens for most clinical cases. However, in recent years, there has been a developing interest in laser- and light-based therapies for acne. A novel treatment in this field is blue light therapy. This system is based on the photosensitivity of porphyrins generated by *Propionibacterium acnes*, the causative agent of acne, to visible light.[43] Protoporphyrin IX absorbs light maximally at 410 nm, which is the wavelength of blue light.[44] Absorption of blue light, in the presence of oxygen molecules, generates singlet oxygen species, which are metastable intermediates that destroy *P. acnes*.[43,45] Furthermore, in vitro studies have found that narrowband blue light diminishes keratinocyte production of IL-1α and ICAM-1, two well-known inflammatory mediators.[43] This finding supports that in addition to bactericidal activity, blue light therapy may also serve to limit inflammation related to acne. In vivo studies conducted with the blue light device Clear Light (CureLight Ltd., Gladstone, New Jersey) reported a 59% to 67% decrease in inflammatory lesions in 80% of patients who had acne, and this effect was maintained for 8 weeks post-treatment.[43] This noteworthy efficacy was also not accompanied by any significant adverse effects, suggesting that blue light therapy may be a safe and reliable treatment for acne.

Lipolysis

Liposuction remains one of the most popular aesthetic procedures performed. Laser-assisted lipolysis was introduced in the early 1990s with the prototype 40 W YAG laser.[46] Although patients reported a reduction in postoperative pain, this device failed to demonstrate a statistically significant improvement over standard liposuction.[46,47] Since then, other laser-assisted liposuction systems have emerged with the aim of delivering more convincing results. Recently, the high energy 1064 nm Nd:YAG laser Smartlipo (Deka, Italy) has demonstrated efficacy in treating focal areas with moderate flaccidity.[47] This system employs a skin-penetrating microcannula that provides direct access to subcutaneous fat.[47] Smartlipo has garnered much attention for its marked ability to induce adipocyte rupture and coagulation of collagen fibers, which are results that cannot be achieved by conventional liposuction. Collagen degeneration and restructuring of the reticular dermis were also observed.[47,48] Furthermore, this device has been associated with decreased bleeding as a result of small vessel coagulation after irradiation.[48] In a recent study of Smartlipo, Kim and Geronemus demonstrated considerable efficacy in treating small areas of undesired fat.[47] In addition to fat reduction, significant dermal tightening overlying the treatment sites was also observed. These results were accompanied by only minor side effects, such as mild bruising, which resolved in 1 to 2 weeks.[47] More studies need to be performed to establish the use of this device for larger areas of fat, which would require higher energy delivery and hence, potentially more complications. Presently, studies indicate that Smartlipo may be a safe and dependable option for treatment of smaller areas, reducing the pain and recovery time associated with conventional liposuction.

Cellulite Treatment

Cellulite, also known as gynoid lipodystrophy, is an aesthetically undesirable problem resulting from an alteration in the architecture of the epidermal-dermal interface.[49] It is much more prevalent in women than men and tends to occur in areas where fat is under the influence of estrogen, such as the hips, thighs, and buttocks.[50] Recent studies have introduced novel applications of technology to treat cellulite. Extracorporeal pulse activation therapy (EPAT) is a noninvasive procedure that improves skin elasticity in patients who have cellulite.[51] Previously, EPAT has been employed to treat a wide assortment of clinical ailments, including musculoskeletal diseases, chronic skin lesions, and kidney stones.[52] EPAT aims to induce tissue damage through the delivery of high pressure acoustic energy; this process is followed by intense dermal remodeling involving the recruitment of chemical mediators, such as vascular endothelial growth factor, endothelial nitric oxide synthase, and heat shock proteins.[51,52] Furthermore, EPAT has been associated with reduced oxidative stress, increased antioxidant production (especially vitamin C), and an upregulation of collagen biosynthesis.[53] These findings have led to studies aimed at investigating the efficacy of EPAT as cellulite treatment. In these studies, EPAT generated a marked increase in skin elasticity, which was maintained six months after treatment.[51] In addition, histologic studies of tissues treated with EPAT have demonstrated neoelastogenesis and neocollagenesis, with a generalized increase in dermal thickness.[52] These encouraging results indicate that EPAT may be a safe and reliable choice for long-lasting treatment of cellulite.

SUMMARY

In recent years, much progress has been made in technological approaches for aesthetic indications. In the area of skin rejuvenation, emerging therapies have not been able to surpass the efficacy demonstrated by conventional ablative lasers. However, the growing demand for safer devices with less down time has led to the development of some innovative therapies. In particular, novel devices combining ablative and fractional modalities exhibit great potential to be future successors. In addition to laser- and light-based therapies, other technologies for varying aesthetic indications have also surfaced with promising results. This trend assures that further advances in science and technology will serve to create superior systems for the aesthetic treatment of skin.

REFERENCES

1. Hantash BM, Renton B, Berkowitz LR, et al. Pilot clinical study of a novel minimally invasive bipolar microneedle radiofrequency device. Lasers Surg Med 2009;41:87–95.

2. Waldorf HA, Kauvar AN, Geronemus RG. Skin resurfacing of fine to deep rhytides using a char-free carbon dioxide laser in 47 patients. Dermatol Surg 1995;21:940–6.

3. Teikemeier G, Goldberg DJ. Skin resurfacing with the erbium:YAG laser. Dermatol Surg 1997;23: 685–7.

4. Sriprachya-Anunt S, Fitzpatrick RE, Goldman MP, et al. Infections complicating pulsed carbon dioxide laser re-surfacing for photoaged facial skin. Dermatol Surg 1997;23:527–35.

5. Lowe NJ, Lask G, Griffin ME. Laser skin resurfacing: pre- and posttreatment guidelines. Dermatol Surg 1995;21:1017–9.

6. Bodendorf MO, Grunewald S, Wetzig T, et al. Fractional laser therapy. J Dtsch Dermatol Ges 2009;7: 301–8.

7. Alster TS. Cutaneous resurfacing with CO_2 and erbium: YAG lasers: preoperative, intraoperative, and postoperative considerations. Plast Reconstr Surg 1999;103:619–32.

8. Kelly KM, Nelson JS, Lask GP, et al. Cryogen spray cooling in combination with nonablative laser treatment of facial rhytides. Arch Dermatol 1999;135: 691–4.

9. Shook BA, Hruza GJ. Periorbital ablative and nonablative re-surfacing. Facial Plast Surg Clin N Am 2005;13:571–82.

10. Hantash BM, Mahmood MB. Fractional photothermolysis: a novel aesthetic laser surgery modality. Dermatol Surg 2007;33:525–34.

11. Boixeda P, Calvo M, Bagazgoitia L. Recent advances in laser therapy and other technologies. Actas Dermosifiliogr 2008;99:262–8.

12. Alster TS. On: increased smooth muscle actin, factor XIIIa, and vimentin-positive cells in the papillary dermis of carbon dioxide laser-debrided porcine skin. Dermatol Surg 1998;24:155.

13. Dang Y, Ren Q, Hoecker S, et al. Biophysical, histological and biochemical changes after non-ablative treatments with the 595 and 1320 nm lasers: a comparative study. Photodermatol Photoimmunol Photomed 2005;21:204–9.

14. Hantash BM, Bedi VP, Sudireddy V, et al. Laser-induced transdermal elimination of dermal component by fractional thermolysis. J Biomed Opt 2006; 11:04115.

15. Karsai S, Raulin. Fractional photothermolysis: a new option for treating melasma? Hautarzt 2008;59: 92–100.

16. Geronemus RG. Fractional photothermolysis: current and future applications. Lasers Surg Med 2006;38:169–76.

17. Alexiades-Armenakas MR, Dover JS, Arndt KA. The spectrum of laser skin resurfacing: non ablative, fractional, and ablative laser resurfacing. J Am Acad Dermatol 2008;58:719–37.

18. Alexiades-Armenakas MR. What is new in lasers and cosmetic procedures from the 2007 AAD annual meeting. J Drugs Dermatol 2007;4:464.

19. Foster KW, Kouba DJ, Fincher EE, et al. Early improvement in rhytides and skin laxity following treatment with a combination fractional laser emitting two wavelengths sequentially. J Drugs Dermatol 2008;2:108–11.

20. Hantash BM, Bedi VP, Chan KF, et al. Ex vivo histological characterization of a novel ablative fractional resurfacing device. Lasers Surg Med 2007;39: 87–95.

21. Goerge T, Peukert N, Bayer H, et al. Ablative fractional photothermolysis – a novel step in skin resurfacing. Med Laser Appl 2008;23:93–8.

22. Hantash BM, Bedi VP, Kapadia B, et al. In vivo histological evaluation of a novel ablative fractional resurfacing device. Lasers Surg Med 2007;39:96–107.

23. Lapidoth M, Yagima Odo M, Odo LM. Novel use of erbium:YAG (2,940-nm) laser for fractional ablative photothermolysis in the treatment of photodamaged facial skin: a pilot study. Dermatol Surg 2008;34: 1048–53.

24. Dierickx CC. The role of deep heating for noninvasive skin rejuvenation. Lasers Surg Med 2006;38: 799–807.

25. Fitzpatrick R, Geronemus R, Goldberg D, et al. Multicenter study of noninvasive radiofrequency for periorbital skin tightening. Lasers Surg Med 2003;33: 232–42.

26. Hsu T, Kaminer MS. The use of nonablative radiofrequency technology to tighten the lower face and neck. Semin Cutan Med Surg 2003;22:115–23.

27. Sadick NS, Alexiades-Armenakas M, Bitter P, et al. Enhanced full-face skin rejuvenation using synchronous intense pulsed optical and conducted bipolar radiofrequency energy (ELOS): introducing selective radio photothermolysis. J Drugs Dermatol 2005;4:181–6.

28. Sadick NS. Bipolar radiofrequency for facial rejuvenation. Facial Plast Surg Clin North Am 2007;15:161–7.

29. Alexiades-Armenakas MR. Rhytides, laxity, and photoaging treated with a combination of radiofrequency, diode laser, and pulsed light and assessed with a comprehensive grading scale. J Drugs Dermatol 2006;5:731–8.

30. Doshi SN, Alster TS. Combination radiofrequency and diode laser for treatment of facial rhytides and skin laxity. J Cosmet Laser Ther 2005;7:11–5.

31. Hantash BM, Ubeid AA, Chang H, et al. Bipolar fractional radiofrequency treatment induces neoelastogenesis and neocollagenesis. Lasers Surg Med 2009;41:1–9 [Epub ahead of print].

32. Laubach HJ, Makin AR, Barthe PG, et al. Intense focused ultrasound: evaluation of a new treatment modality for precise microcoagulation within the skin. Dermatol Surg 2008;34:727–34.

33. Rabkin BA, Zderic V, Vaezy S. Hyperecho in ultrasound images of HIFU therapy: involvement of cavitation. Ultrasound Med Biol 2005;31:947–56.

34. Van Leenders GJ, Beerlage HP, Ruijter ET, et al. Histopathological changes associated with high intensity focused ultrasound (HIFU) treatment for localised adenocarcinoma of the prostate. J Clin Pathol 2000;53:391–4.

35. Chapelon JY, Ribault M, Vernier F, et al. Treatment of localised prostate cancer with transrectal high intensity focused ultrasound. Eur J Ultrasound 1999;9:31–8.

36. Goss SA, Johnston RL, Dunn F. Comprehensive compilation of empirical ultrasonic properties of mammalian tissues. J Acoust Soc Am 1978;64:423–57.

37. Grimes PE. Microdermabrasion. Dermatol Surg 2006;31:1160–5.

38. Clark C. New directions in skin care. Clin Plast Surg 2001;28:745–50.

39. Savardekar P. Microdermabrasion. Indian J Dermatol Venereol Leprol 2007;73:277–9.

40. Karimipour DJ, Kang S, Johnson TM, et al. Microdermabrasion: a molecular analysis following a single treatment. J Am Acad Dermatol 2005;52:215–23.

41. Karimipour DJ, Kang S, Johnson TM, et al. Microdermabrasion with and without aluminum oxide crystal abrasion: a comparative molecular analysis of dermal remodeling. J Am Acad Dermatol 2006;54:405–10.

42. Munavalli GS, Weiss RA. Evidence for laser- and light-based treatment of acne vulgaris. Semin Cutan Med Surg 2008;27:207–11.

43. Taub AF. Procedural treatments for acne vulgaris. Dermtol Surg 2007;33:1005–26.

44. Kalka K, Merk H, Mukhtar H. Photodynamic therapy in dermatology. J Am Acad Dermatol 2000;42:389–413.

45. Weishaupt K, Gomer C, Dougherty T. Identification of singlet oxygen as the cytotoxic agent in photoinactivation of a murine tumor. Cancer Res 1976;36:2326–9.

46. Mann MW, Palm MD, Sengelmann RD. New advances in liposuction technology. Semin Cutan Med Surg 2008;27:72–82.

47. Kim KH, Geronemus RG. Laser lipolysis using a Novel 1,064 nm Nd:YAG Laser. Dermatol Surg 2006;32:241–8.

48. Goldman A, Schavelzon DE, Blugerman GS. Laser-lipolysis: liposuction using Nd:YAG laser. Rev Soc Bras Cir Plast 2002;17:17–26.

49. Quatresooz P, Xhauflaire-Uhoda E, Piérard-Franchimont C, et al. Cellulite histopathology and related mechanobiology. Int J Cosmet Sci 2006;28:207–10.

50. Goldman A, Gotkin RH, Sarnoff DS, et al. Cellulite: a new treatment approach combining subdermal Nd:YAG laser lipolysis and autologous fat transplantation. Aesthet Surg J 2008;28:656–62.

51. Christ C, Brenke R, Sattler G, et al. Improvement in skin elasticity in the treatment of cellulite and connective tissue weakness by means of extracorporeal pulse activation therapy. Aesthet Surg J 2008;28:538–44.

52. Kuhn C, Angehrn F, Sonnabend O, et al. Impact of extracorporeal shock waves on the human skin with cellulite: a case study of an unique instance. Clin Interv Aging 2008;3:201–10.

53. Ku Siems W, Grune T, Voss P, et al. Anti-fibrosclerotic effects of shock wave therapy in lipedema and cellulite. Biofactors 2005;24:275–82.

Skin Type Classification Systems Old and New

Wendy E. Roberts, MD, FAAD

KEYWORDS
- Cosmetic skin type • Classification systems
- Cosmetic outcomes

The observation that skin of any color has a unique response when under environmental or physical stress dates past antiquity to ancient civilizations, including Egyptian, Mayan, Aboriginal, and Indian. These cultures, understanding their individual skin qualities, would cover, protect, embellish, and manipulate the skin to their advantage. In some ancient cultures the development of skin laxity and keloid formation is considered desirable and beautiful. In the dawn of Western medicine the predominant skin type was light/white in color and procedures and treatments were geared toward that one phenotype. There was not a perceived need to classify the different types of Caucasian skin because there were little observed differences in clinical behavior among the European skin type of that time. As we look ahead, modern-day globalization has impacted on every aspect of life, including our human phenotype. The world population has grown to 6.7 billion people.[1] Mixing of ethnicities has led to the increased emergence of mixed genotypes resultant from interethnic and interracial marriages and progeny. According to Taylor, United States intermarriage patterns as of 1998 reveal 9% white/black intermarriage rates; 19% white/Asian; 12% white/Native American; 52% white/Hispanic; and the remaining 7% involving other admixtures.[2] This mixing of ethnicities leads to a significant change in the world demographics as we continue to evolve and diversify at unprecedented levels. We are developing new skin types at a rapid rate. The US Census Bureau statistics in 1990 list six races with 23 racial subtypes. Ten years later, the 2000 Census statistics show the same six race categories with 67subtypes.[3] It is becoming increasingly apparent that the world composition includes many variations and combinations of traditional skin types. Ethnic people of various skin colors now compose one third of the standing 306 million people in the United States and 6.1 million are combinations of two or more races.[4] The emerging world phenotype continues to have far-reaching, important implications for patients and those involved in caring for the skin. We have all experienced the phenotypically blonde-haired, blue-eyed patient that develops scarring after cosmetic surgery and conversely the olive-complexioned patient who has no adverse sequelae from a deep trichloroacetic acid (TCA) peel. How do we communicate the subtleties of different skin types? How do we determine who is at risk from a certain cosmetic procedure and predict reactions? How do we classify homogenous and mixed skin types and design our treatment protocols for best outcomes? How do we build on the rich knowledge of skin type needed for future growth? Globalization affects the skin-care industry as the invention of skin-oriented products, which are not only efficacious but targeted toward specific skin types, becomes a necessity. The ability to be used safely and effectively in every skin color is quickly becoming the gold standard in laser and light technology.

There are several unfavorable reactions that may result in skin of any color that undergoes a cosmetic procedure. Chemical peels, Intense Pulsed Light (IPL), and hair removal laser are some of the more commonly performed cosmetic procedures that have produced untoward complications. There are certain skin types that are at greater risk than others for development of one or more of these procedures. Performing these procedures in mixed and global skin types

Desert Dermatology Skin Institute, 72301 Country Club Drive, Suite 101, Rancho Mirage, CA 922701, USA
E-mail address: drwerderm@aol.com

Dermatol Clin 27 (2009) 529–533
doi:10.1016/j.det.2009.08.006
0733-8635/09/$ – see front matter © 2009 Published by Elsevier Inc.

requires an understanding of the nuances of skin color and they should not be taken without advanced training. The most common complications from skin injury and insult are hyperpigmentation, hypopigmentation, scarring, and keloid formation. There is an important medical need regarding the health of patients to determine the skin effects from procedural and cosmetic dermatology. The goal is to identify these risks for patients and avoid complications. Increased mixed skin types enter our offices and the world of procedural and cosmetic dermatology. It is our goal to assist them in the best clinical outcomes, which includes factoring in their skin type into the planning of periprocedural period and the post-care. There remains an interest in classifying skin types and skin responses and the literature to date is reviewed.

THE FITZPATRICK SCALE

Developed in 1975, the landmark Fitzpatrick scale offers a useful method of classifying patients' skin phototype, and thus, the ability to burn and tan when challenged with UV radiation (UVR). In determining the phototype, the emphasis was placed on the color of the skin and eyes and the ability of that skin to burn or tan. Initially established as a four-point scale and in 1988 modified to include darker skin tones (types V and VI), Fitzpatrick is most commonly used to determine the skin's response to UVR and the skin's ability to tan.[5] This skin phototype has been used synonymously as a skin type within the dermatologic community. However, Fitzpatrick scores do little to predict the skin's response to trauma from certain procedures, such as laser and surgery. In addition, the Fitzpatrick system is potentially misleading because all skin types, even those classified as Fitzpatrick types V and VI, are susceptible to some element of burning from UVR. The clinical corollary is that we have now evolved to recommend UVR protection for all skin types including the darkest of skin. This system however remains the gold standard of classification systems.

KAWADA SKIN CLASSIFICATION SYSTEM (1986)

UV-B–induced erythema, delayed tanning, and UV-A–induced immediate tanning in the Japanese were investigated on the skin of the backs of 65 healthy subjects. The subjects were classified according to Japanese skin type, based on personal history of sun reactivity. This system is useful, but limited to Japanese individuals.[6]

THE GLOGAU SCALE (1994)

The Glogau Scale classifies the degree of photoaging and categorizes the amount of wrinkling and discoloration in patients' skin.[7] While undeniably useful, the Glogau system does not address the signs of photoaging in mixed ethnic-racial skin types, which may include various pigmentary dyschromias, midfacial decent, and periorbital darkening.

LANCER ETHNICITY SCALE (1998)

The Lancer ethnicity scale is a classification system that looked at ancestry and Fitzpatrick skin types in the calculation of healing efficacy and times in cosmetic patients undergoing laser or chemical peeling.[8]

GOLDMAN WORLD CLASSIFICATION OF SKIN TYPE (2002)

This classification system was developed to examine various skin color responses to burning, tanning, and postinflammatory pigmentation.[9]

FANOUS CLASSIFICATION (2002)

Fanous classification is a classification system for laser resurfacing, chemical peels, and dermabrasion. This system is based on racial-genetic origins and describes six subraces and discusses the evaluation of patients.[10]

WILLIS AND EARLES SCALE (2005)

The Willis and Earles scale was a proposal for a new skin classification system relevant to people of African descent that only classifies skin color, reaction to UV light, and association of pigmentary disorders.[11]

THE TAYLOR HYPERPIGMENTATION SCALE (2006)

The Taylor hyperpigmentation scale is a visual hyperpigmentation scale developed in May 2006, which consists of laminated cards that have 10 to 15 skin hues and up to 100 gradations of different colors of pigmentation. An area of hyperpigmentation is matched to the card color. This scale evaluates lesions of dyschromia.[12]

THE BAUMANN SKIN TYPE SOLUTION (2006)

The Bauman skin type solution was introduced and popularized in the book, *Skin Type Solution,* which profiles 16 common skin types. This system is used primarily by consumers as a guide to proper skin-care techniques for various complexions. It does not aim to predict outcomes.[13]

THE ROBERTS HYPERPIGMENTATION SCALE

The Roberts hyperpigmentation scale (H) is a seven-point system that measures the natural history of postinflammatory pigmentation in an individual and the likelihood to incur a pigmentation problem. One individual may experience hypo- and hyperpigmentation and should be scored for both. This value is based on past medical history, clinical examination, and ancestral background. This scale is particularly important given the rapid rate of ethnic and racial diversification throughout the world.[14]

THE ROBERTS SCARRING SCALE

The Roberts scarring scale (S) is a six-point scale that classifies patients' patterns of scarring. An individual's score on the scarring scale helps to determine short- and long-term effects of numerous medical treatments and procedures. Patients should be scored to communicate the worst response they have had. Though history is helpful, a complete skin examination would be most thorough as a scar may be forgotten when verbally reported.[14]

In the aforementioned classification systems there was no single system that captured the essential factors that determine outcomes from environmental insult, such as trauma, procedural dermatology, and plastic surgery.

There was a need to create a tool that could be used to communicate the very important message of how an individual's skin responds to insult, injury, and inflammation. This tool should be able to be used for all skin types while being especially useful for identifying the inherent needs, risks, and propensities of mixed ethnic and racial skin types. This tool would be used to select and plan cosmetic and medical procedures, manage wound care and skin repair, aid in selecting appropriate skin-care products, and most importantly, assist in avoiding potential complications from any procedure that involves the skin, whether a basic comedo extraction or a laser-resurfacing procedure.

THE ROBERTS SKIN TYPE CLASSIFICATION SYSTEM

To determine a patient's profile using the Roberts Skin Type Classification System the clinician should first refer to **Box 1** and familiarize themselves with the listed scales that were reviewed earlier. There are four elements and each element gets assigned a numeric value or feature.[14] The

---

Box 1
Four elements of the Robert's skin type classification system

Fitzpatrick (FZ) scale (measures skin phototypes)

Type FZI white skin, always burns, never tans

Type FZII white skin, always burns, minimal tan

Type FZIII white skin, burns minimally, tans moderately and gradually

Type FZIV light brown skin, burns minimally, tans well

Type FZV brown skin, rarely burns, tans deeply

Type FZVI dark brown/black skin, never burns, tans deeply

Robert's hyperpigmentation (H) scale (measures propensity for pigmentation)

Type H0 hypopigmentation

Type HI minimal and transient (<1 year) hyperpigmentation

Type HII minimal and permanent (>1 year) hyperpigmentation

Type HIII moderate and transient (<1 year) hyperpigmentation

Type HIV moderate and permanent (>1 year) hyperpigmentation

Type HV severe and transient (<1 year) hyperpigmentation

Type HVI severe and permanent (>1 year) hyperpigmentation

Glogau (G) scale (describes photoaging)

Type GI no wrinkles, early photoaging

Type GII wrinkles in motion, early to moderate photoaging

Type GIII wrinkles at rest, advanced photoaging

Type GIV only wrinkles, severe photoaging

Roberts scarring (S) scale (scar morphology)

Type S0 atrophy

Type SI none

Type SII macule

Type SIII plaque within scar boundaries

Type SIV keloid

Type SV keloidal nodule

Table 1	
Robert's skin classification system	
Element	Feature (Value)
Fitzpatrick phototype	FZ (types 1–6)
Roberts hyperpigmentation	H (types 0–6)
Glogau photoaging	G (types 1–5)
Roberts scarring	S (types 0–5)

Each element, with its companion feature (numeric value), is placed in a serial format (ie, *FZx, Hx, Gx, Sx*).

assignment is straightforward and based on hin scan boundaries (**Table 1**).

This profile results in a specific classification of a skin type for patients of any color or mix of colors. This system is not color dependant. It functions as a system for all skin types and can classify anyone from anywhere in the world.

To define patients' individualized skin-type profile using the Roberts Skin Type Classification System, the clinician conducts a physical examination, performs a complete visual review of the skin, gathers historical information, such as ancestry, history of pigmentation, and scarring, and when necessary, evaluates test site reactions to assign a feature to the four elements according to the guidelines for each. Once a clinician establishes a profile using the four-part Roberts System, the data can be used to determine the safest and most efficacious treatment plan based on the patients' likely response to injury, insult, and inflammation. Patients may carry this designation similar to a blood type and use it as a means of communication, when necessary, to identify procedural or environmental risks.

Clinical Patient Example #1

A 30-year-old woman of Indian and English descent is interested in IPL, and would like to know if she is a good candidate for the procedure.

> She, per history, burns minimally and tans well (FZ4)
> She has, per history, moderate and transient hyperpigmentation, but postinflammatory hyperpigmentation (PIH) is also noted on skin examination of old acne sites (H3)
> She has early photoaging (G1)
> She has two hypertrophic scars (S3) also seen on skin examination
> Roberts Skin Type profile: FZ4, H3, G1, S3

The clinical response included the following: Given her Roberts skin type profile, this individual is not a candidate for IPL. Despite her English heritage, her H3 score on the hyperpigmentation scale and S3 score on the scarring scale informs the clinician that she would be a possible risk for PIH and scarring as a result of the procedure. One possible option would be to proceed with a low IPL setting, but the low setting may not achieve the effect the patient desires and she would end up being dissatisfied. Select another procedure for her chief complaint.

Clinical Patient Example #2

A 50-year-old Caucasian woman is referred for excision of a presternal nevus and on physical examination has an abdominal hypertrophic scar. Her Roberts skin type profile is: FZ1, H1, G3, S3. The clinical response includes the following: Given the patient's Roberts skin type profile and the location of the nevus, she is at possible risk for a scar in a highly visible location. Despite her light white complexion she has a propensity to scar, which is determined by history and skin examination. When this is discussed with the patient she decides to keep the benign nevus versus risk an unsightly scar on her décolleté.

SUMMARY

The history of classifying skin types is rather new and there has been considerable progress made with continuing awareness. The Fitzpatrick Skin Phototype Classification remains the gold standard. It is simple and user friendly, however, this system fails to accurately predict skin reactions. The Roberts Skin Type Classification System is a tool to predict the skin response to injury and insult from dermatologic and cosmetic procedures and identify the propensity of sequelae from inflammatory skin disorders. It can be a predictor of an impending complication, such as hyperpigmentation and scarring, which can then be avoided. In addition, it includes the skin phototype and photoage. In evaluating patients' skin and developing a cosmetic plan the four indices outlined in this article, hyper/hypopigmentation risk, scarring risk, skin phototype, and photoage are crucial to identify for optimal outcomes. This system will keep relevant with evolving race and world composition, and will function as a tool for description and communication throughout the scientific community. It can serve as a universal language used by physicians and the skin-care specialty to classify, evaluate, and properly treat patients' skin types anywhere in the world. Equipped with this standardized methodology for identifying and assessing different skin types, dermatologists and plastic surgeons can increase the effectiveness of patients' evaluation and assure the highest level of safety and benefits of patients' treatments for our emerging world phenotype.

REFERENCES

1. Population Reference Bureau 2009. Availabel at: www.PRB.org. Accessed October 5, 2009.
2. Taylor SC. Skin of color: biology, structure, function, and implications for dermatologic disease. J Am Acad Dermatol 2002;46(2):S41–62.
3. US census bureau 1990, 2000, Available at: www.census.gov/. Accessed March 01, 2008.
4. Wikipedia Demographics of the United States. Available at: http://en.wikipedia.org/wiki/Demographics_of_the_United_States. Accessed October 5, 2009.
5. Fitzpatrick TB. The validity and practicality of sunreactive skin types I-VI. Arch Dermatol 1988;124:869–71.
6. Kawada A. UVB-induced erythema, delayed tanning, and UVA-induced immediate tanning in Japanese skin. Photodermatol 1986;3:327–33.
7. Glogau RG. Chemical peeling and aging skin. J Geriatr Dermatol 1994;12:31.
8. Lancer HA. Lancer Ethnicity Scale (LES) [letter]. Lasers Surg Med 1998;22:9.
9. Goldman M. Universal classification of skin type. J Cosmet Dermatol 2002;15:53–4, 57.
10. Fanous N. A new patient classification for laser resurfacing and peels. Aesthetic Plast Surg 26:99–104.
11. Willis I, Earles MR. A new classification system relevant to people of African Descent. J Cosmet Dermatol 2005;18(3):209–16.
12. Taylor SC, Westerhof W, Im S, et al. Noninvasive techniques for the evaluation of skin color. J Am Acad Dermatol 2006;54:S282–90.
13. Baumann L. Skin type solution. Available at: www.skintypesolutions.com/. Accessed March 2009.
14. Roberts WE. The Roberts skin type classification system. J Drugs Dermatol 2008;7(5):452–6.

Index

Note: Page numbers of article titles are in **boldface** type.

0733-8635/09/$ – see front matter © 2009 Elsevier Inc. All rights reserved.

United States Postal Service

Statement of Ownership, Management, and Circulation
(All Periodicals Publications Except Requestor Publications)

1. Publication Title	2. Publication Number	3. Filing Date
Dermatologic Clinics of North America	0 0 0 - 7 0 5	9/15/09

4. Issue Frequency	5. Number of Issues Published Annually	6. Annual Subscription Price
Jan, Apr, Jul, Oct	4	$274.00

7. Complete Mailing Address of Known Office of Publication (Not printer) (Street, city, county, state, and ZIP+4®)

Contact Person
Stephen Bushing

Elsevier Inc.
360 Park Avenue South
New York, NY 10010-1710

Telephone (Include area code)
215-239-3688

8. Complete Mailing Address of Headquarters or General Business Office of Publisher (Not printer)

Elsevier Inc., 360 Park Avenue South, New York, NY 10010-1710

9. Full Names and Complete Mailing Addresses of Publisher, Editor, and Managing Editor (Do not leave blank)

Publisher (Name and complete mailing address)

John Schrefer , Elsevier, Inc., 1600 John F. Kennedy Blvd. Suite 1800, Philadelphia, PA 19103-2899

Editor (Name and complete mailing address)

Carla Holloway-Elsevier, Inc., 1600 John F. Kennedy Blvd. Suite 1800, Philadelphia, PA 19103-2899

Managing Editor (Name and complete mailing address)

Catherine Bewick, Elsevier, Inc., 1600 John F. Kennedy Blvd. Suite 1800, Philadelphia, PA 19103-2899

10. Owner (Do not leave blank. If the publication is owned by a corporation, give the name and address of the corporation immediately followed by the names and addresses of all stockholders owning or holding 1 percent or more of the total amount of stock. If not owned by a corporation, give the names and addresses of the individual owners. If owned by a partnership or other unincorporated firm, give its name and address as well as those of each individual owner. If the publication is published by a nonprofit organization, give its name and address.)

Full Name	Complete Mailing Address
Wholly owned subsidiary of	4520 East-West Highway
Reed/Elsevier, US holdings	Bethesda, MD 20814

11. Known Bondholders, Mortgagees, and Other Security Holders Owning or Holding 1 Percent or More of Total Amount of Bonds, Mortgages, or Other Securities. If none, check box ☐ None

Full Name	Complete Mailing Address
N/A	

12. Tax Status (For completion by nonprofit organizations authorized to mail at nonprofit rates) (Check one)
The purpose, function, and nonprofit status of this organization and the exempt status for federal income tax purposes:
☐ Has Not Changed During Preceding 12 Months
☐ Has Changed During Preceding 12 Months (Publisher must submit explanation of change with this statement)

PS Form 3526, September 2007 (Page 1 of 3 (Instructions Page 3)) PSN 7530-01-000-9931 PRIVACY NOTICE: See our Privacy policy in www.usps.com

13. Publication Title	14. Issue Date for Circulation Data Below
Dermatologic Clinics of North America	July 2009

15. Extent and Nature of Circulation		Average No. Copies Each Issue During Preceding 12 Months	No. Copies of Single Issue Published Nearest to Filing Date
a. Total Number of Copies (Net press run)		1254	1200
b. Paid Circulation (By Mail and Outside the Mail)	(1) Mailed Outside-County Paid Subscriptions Stated on PS Form 3541. (Include paid distribution above nominal rate, advertiser's proof copies, and exchange copies)	452	416
	(2) Mailed In-County Paid Subscriptions Stated on PS Form 3541 (Include paid distribution above nominal rate, advertiser's proof copies, and exchange copies)		
	(3) Paid Distribution Outside the Mails Including Sales Through Dealers and Carriers, Street Vendors, Counter Sales, and Other Paid Distribution Outside USPS®	252	244
	(4) Paid Distribution by Other Classes Mailed Through the USPS (e.g. First-Class Mail®)		
c. Total Paid Distribution (Sum of 15b (1), (2), (3), and (4))	▲	704	660
d. Free or Nominal Rate Distribution (By Mail and Outside the Mail)	(1) Free or Nominal Rate Outside-County Copies Included on PS Form 3541	85	86
	(2) Free or Nominal Rate In-County Copies Included on PS Form 3541		
	(3) Free or Nominal Rate Copies Mailed at Other Classes Through the USPS (e.g. First-Class Mail)		
	(4) Free or Nominal Rate Distribution Outside the Mail (Carriers or other means)		
e. Total Free or Nominal Rate Distribution (Sum of 15d (1), (2), (3) and (4))	▲	85	86
f. Total Distribution (Sum of 15c and 15e)	▲	789	746
g. Copies not Distributed (See instructions to publishers #4 (page #3))	▲	465	454
h. Total (Sum of 15f and g)	▲	1254	1200
i. Percent Paid (15c divided by 15f times 100)		89.23%	88.47%

16. Publication of Statement of Ownership

☐ If the publication is a general publication, publication of this statement is required. Will be printed in the October 2009 issue of this publication. ☐ Publication not required

17. Signature and Title of Editor, Publisher, Business Manager, or Owner	Date
[signature] Stephen R. Bushing – Subscription Services Coordinator	September 15, 2009

I certify that all information furnished on this form is true and complete. I understand that anyone who furnishes false or misleading information on this form or who omits material or information requested on the form may be subject to criminal sanctions (including fines and imprisonment) and/or civil sanctions (including civil penalties).

PS Form 3526, September 2007 (Page 2 of 3)

Moving?

Make sure your subscription moves with you!

To notify us of your new address, find your **Clinics Account Number** (located on your mailing label above your name), and contact customer service at:

Email: journalscustomerservice-usa@elsevier.com

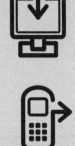

800-654-2452 (subscribers in the U.S. & Canada)
314-447-8871 (subscribers outside of the U.S. & Canada)

Fax number: 314-447-8029

Elsevier Health Sciences Division
Subscription Customer Service
3251 Riverport Lane
Maryland Heights, MO 63043

*To ensure uninterrupted delivery of your subscription, please notify us at least 4 weeks in advance of move.

ELSEVIER